Page #	Name of Drug / Med	Page #	
1		26	
2		27	
3		28	
4		29	
5		30	
6		31	
7		32	
8		33	
9		34	
10		35	
11		36	
12		37	
13		38	
14		39	
15		40	
16		41	
17		42	
18		43	
19		44	
20		45	
21		46	
22		47	
23		48	
24		49	
25		50	

Page #	Name of Drug / Med	Page #	Name of Drug / Med
51		76	
52		77	
53		78	
54		79	
55		80	
56		81	
57		82	
58		83	
59		84	
60		85	
61		86	
62		87	
63		88	
64		89	
65		90	
66		91	
67		92	
68		93	
69		94	
70		95	
71		96	
72		97	
73		98	
74		99	
75		100	

Page #	Name of Drug / Med	Page #	Name of Drug / Med
101		126	
102		127	
103		128	
104		129	
105		130	
106		131	
107		132	
108		133	
109		134	
110		135	
111		136	
112		137	
113		138	
114		139	
115		140	
116		141	
117		142	
118		143	
119		144	
120		145	
121		146	
122		147	
123		148	
124		149	
125		150	

Controlled Substance Record Book (CSRB)
- Instructions -

A Controlled Substance Record Book (CSRB) will be used to log and count all controlled drugs / medications. There will be a CSRB at each location where controlled substances are maintained. The CSRB location including county, building, and clinic location, and start and end dates of all records will be included on the *RECORD BOOK STATUS* page and spine of each CSRB. CSRBs will not be transferred between locations.

1. **Receipt of Controlled Substances (Drugs / Medications)**
   a. Enter drug / medication item on the *INDEX PAGE* of the CSRB in the next available line that corresponds to the next *CONTROLLED DRUG / MED SUPPLY* page in the CSRB. DO NOT leave any blank lines.
   b. For stock drugs / medications: include drug name and strength.
   c. For patient specific drugs / medications: include drug name, strength, patient name, and ID #.
   d. Enter drug / medication item on the next available *CONTROLLED DRUG / MED SUPPLY* page in the CSRB. Complete all information at the top of the page. DO NOT leave any blank pages.

2. **Administration / Use of Controlled Drugs / Medications**
   a. Each drug / medication dose will be accounted for at the time of the administration, including the date and time administered, amount used, remaining supply, the patient name, and the Nurse / Licensed Professional (*hereinafter referred to in this record book as "Nurse/LP"*) signatures.
   b. Administration of each drug / medication must also be documented in the patient's personal Medication Administration Record (MAR).

3. **Destruction / Waste of Controlled Drugs / Medications**
   a. Destruction / waste of any amount of a controlled drug / medication must be witnessed.
   b. Wastage must be entered on the *CONTROLLED DRUG / MED SUPPLY* page- on the line corresponding to the date and time the drug / med was signed out, along with both signatures of the Nurse/LPs.
   c. Drugs / medications are to be made irretrievable- crush and mix with a small amount of water to make a slurry, then pour into the drug / medication disposal bin for collection and incineration.
   d. All records regarding destruction / waste must be maintained on-site for a minimum of 5 years.

4. **Shift Counting of Controlled Drugs / Medications**
   a. All counts will be documented on the *SHIFT COUNT – CONTROLLED DRUGS / MEDS* pages.
   b. Counts for any controlled drugs / medications that are not accessed daily (secured back up stock, for example) will, at a minimum, be completed and documented weekly by 2 Nurse/LPs.
   c. Every shift the Nurse/LP going off duty will count with the Nurse/LP coming on duty.
   d. The Date and Time the count was completed will be added to the first available line on the page. No lines will be left blank or skipped for any reason.
   e. Both Nurse/LPs will verify the physical amount on hand corresponds to the amount recorded as *Present Balance* on each active *CONTROLLED DRUG / MED SUPPLY* page.
   f. The count will be marked as correct or incorrect. If a count is incorrect, the *Error in End of Shift Narcotic Count Form* (not in this CSRB) will be completed by both Nurse/LPs and notification provided to the Program Manager / Health Service Administrator / Director of Nursing.
   g. Both Nurse/LPs completing the count will sign, not initial, the count.

5. **Transfer of Controlled Drugs / Medications to a New Page**
   a. When a *CONTROLLED DRUG / MED SUPPLY* page is completed, the information must be transferred to a new page. Locate the next available page (DO NOT skip any pages) in the current CSRB and enter the information as indicated in "Receipt of Controlled Substances" (see #1 above), including the page from which the drug / medication was transferred.
   b. Fold over the completed page & complete the information in the *TRANSFER TO NEW PAGE* Section.

6. **Transfer of Controlled Drugs / Medications to a New / Different Location**
    a. When a drug / medication is transferred to another location, it must be removed from the current CSRB and entered in the CSRB at the location to which it is being transferred.
    b. Enter a line through any rows not used on the *CONTROLLED DRUG / MED SUPPLY* page.
    c. Fold over the page and complete the information in the *TRANSFER TO DIFFERENT LOCATION* Section. Enter the book location and page number to which the count is being transferred, including the signature of both Nurse/LPs making the transfer, if possible.
    d. Enter the drug / medication in the new CSRB as indicated in "Receipt of Controlled Substances" (see #1 above). Both Nurse/LPs should sign the entry into the new location, if possible.

7. **Transfer of all Controlled Drugs / Medications to a New Book**
    a. When a CSRB is full and it becomes necessary to transfer the medication from one CSRB to another, follow the directions as indicated in "Transferring Medication to a Different Location" (see #6c-d above (including the reference to #1 above)).
    b. Enter the "End Date" on the CSRB spine and the *RECORD BOOK STATUS* page. Deliver the full (completed) CSRB to the appropriate person for archival / storage as required by law.

8. **Surrender of Controlled Drugs / Medications to a Person**
    a. In the event a patient is admitted with a controlled drug / medication / other item and it becomes the responsibility of the healthcare unit, log the drug / medication / other item into the CSRB as indicated in "Receipt of Controlled Substances" (see #1 above).
    b. Upon release from the facility the patient's personal property may be released to him / her, provided the prescribed drug(s) / medication(s) / other item(s) have not expired.
    c. Enter a line through any remaining rows on the *CONTROLLED DRUG / MED SUPPLY* page.
    d. Fold over the page and complete the information in the *SURRENDER TO PERSON* section.
    e. Add any additional pertinent information next to the section including the relationship and purpose of surrender.
    f. The person receiving the drug / medication / other item, as well as the person surrendering the drug / medication / other item must both sign the *SURRENDER TO PERSON* section.

9. **Records Retention (all controlled substance records must be maintained for a minimum of 5 years):**
    a. Pharmacy manifests that list controlled medications sent to site.
    b. Completed Controlled Substance Record Books (CSRBs).
    c. DEA Destruction certificates for any medications destroyed on site.

Helpful Hints:

1. If the site only has one locked narcotic box there should be only one active CSRB for that box.

2. There should only be one current active *CONTROLLED DRUG / MED SUPPLY* page for each stock drug / medication. For example: if the site receives 3 cards of Valium 10mg, the entire 90 pills are entered on one page with the starting count of 90. When the page is completed then transfer the remaining amount to the next available page in the CSRB. Fold the page over to complete the transfer section and make it easier to skip past that page during shift counts.

3. If a patient receives 2 pills at one time you do not have to use 2 lines to sign off 2 doses, just use one line and indicate 2 pills were given.

4. Each different strength of a drug / medication requires a different *CONTROLLED DRUG / MED SUPPLY* page. For example, Valium 5mg and Valium 10mg tabs should be on two different pages.

5. If access to drugs / medications / supplies is STRICTLY limited to a single individual (for example, in an office) then those drugs / medications / supplies need only be counted once weekly, but two Nurse/LPs are required to complete the count (see #4b above).

Controlled Substance Record Book

(Blue Cover)

Printed in the Unites States of America
First Printing: September 2017
ISBN: 978-1975960780

This publication is designed to provide accurate and relative information in regard to the subject matter covered. It is designed to be generic in its use and application. All users must understand and apply the applicable policies, procedures, laws, statutes, regulations, and all other requirements regarding the subject matter hereof. It is sold "as is" with the understanding that neither the author nor the publisher is engaged in rendering medical, legal, or other professional services. If medical or legal advice or other expert assistance is required, the services of a competent professional person should be sought.

A production of: MAXnJAX Media & BLAST Information Systems

For more information please visit: MAXnJAX.com/substancebook

- Order Copies -
www.maxnjax.com/substancebook
email us at: info@maxnjax.com
amazon.com, using the ISBN number above
(visit our web site for special offers)

Need a specific form or layout? Want a customized look or color scheme? Want to include your company name, logo, pictures, graphics, etc.? Send an email with your request and we will work with you to provide an affordable option to meet your individual needs.

- RECORD BOOK STATUS -

Book Location
(i.e. station, cart, etc.)

_____

Book Identifier / Number / Code
(i.e. use a distinctive identifier, number, code, etc.)

_____

Book Start Date

_____ / _____ / _____

Transferred From Book: _____

Book End Date

_____ / _____ / _____

Transferred To Book: _____

- OTHER INFORMATION -

Issued To:	

Signature:	**Date:**	
Issued By:	**Date:**	
Phone #:	**Cell #:**	
Email(s):		
Other:		

Company / Group:			
Department:			
Address 1:			
Address 2:			
City:	**State:**	**Zip:**	
Other:			

Notes:

SHIFT COUNT – CONTROLLED DRUGS / MEDS

Today's Date	Time Of Day	Signature of Nurse/LP Going Off Duty	Signature of Nurse/LP Coming On Duty	Count Correct?	
				Yes	No

At each shift change, all controlled drugs / meds must be counted.
Complete *Report of Error in End of Shift Narcotic Count Form* to document any discrepancies.

SHIFT COUNT – CONTROLLED DRUGS / MEDS

Today's Date	Time Of Day	Signature of Nurse/LP Going Off Duty	Signature of Nurse/LP Coming On Duty	Count Correct?	
				Yes	No

At each shift change, all controlled drugs / meds must be counted.
Complete *Report of Error in End of Shift Narcotic Count Form* to document any discrepancies.

SHIFT COUNT – CONTROLLED DRUGS / MEDS

Today's Date	Time Of Day	Signature of Nurse/LP Going Off Duty	Signature of Nurse/LP Coming On Duty	Count Correct?	
				Yes	No

At each shift change, all controlled drugs / meds must be counted.
Complete *Report of Error in End of Shift Narcotic Count Form* to document any discrepancies.

SHIFT COUNT – CONTROLLED DRUGS / MEDS

Today's Date	Time Of Day	Signature of Nurse/LP Going Off Duty	Signature of Nurse/LP Coming On Duty	Count Correct?	
				Yes	No

At each shift change, all controlled drugs / meds must be counted.
Complete *Report of Error in End of Shift Narcotic Count Form* to document any discrepancies.

SHIFT COUNT – CONTROLLED DRUGS / MEDS

Today's Date	Time Of Day	Signature of Nurse/LP Going Off Duty	Signature of Nurse/LP Coming On Duty	Count Correct?	
				Yes	No

At each shift change, all controlled drugs / meds must be counted.
Complete *Report of Error in End of Shift Narcotic Count Form* to document any discrepancies.

SHIFT COUNT – CONTROLLED DRUGS / MEDS

Today's Date	Time Of Day	Signature of Nurse/LP Going Off Duty	Signature of Nurse/LP Coming On Duty	Count Correct?	
				Yes	No

At each shift change, all controlled drugs / meds must be counted.
Complete *Report of Error in End of Shift Narcotic Count Form* to document any discrepancies.

SHIFT COUNT – CONTROLLED DRUGS / MEDS

Today's Date	Time Of Day	Signature of Nurse/LP Going Off Duty	Signature of Nurse/LP Coming On Duty	Count Correct?	
				Yes	No

At each shift change, all controlled drugs / meds must be counted.
Complete *Report of Error in End of Shift Narcotic Count Form* to document any discrepancies.

SHIFT COUNT – CONTROLLED DRUGS / MEDS

Today's Date	Time Of Day	Signature of Nurse/LP Going Off Duty	Signature of Nurse/LP Coming On Duty	Count Correct?	
				Yes	No

At each shift change, all controlled drugs / meds must be counted.
Complete *Report of Error in End of Shift Narcotic Count Form* to document any discrepancies.

SHIFT COUNT – CONTROLLED DRUGS / MEDS

Today's Date	Time Of Day	Signature of Nurse/LP Going Off Duty	Signature of Nurse/LP Coming On Duty	Count Correct?	
				Yes	No

At each shift change, all controlled drugs / meds must be counted.
Complete *Report of Error in End of Shift Narcotic Count Form* to document any discrepancies.

SHIFT COUNT – CONTROLLED DRUGS / MEDS

Today's Date	Time Of Day	Signature of Nurse/LP Going Off Duty	Signature of Nurse/LP Coming On Duty	Count Correct?	
				Yes	No

At each shift change, all controlled drugs / meds must be counted.
Complete *Report of Error in End of Shift Narcotic Count Form* to document any discrepancies.

Today's Date	Time Of Day	Signature of Nurse/LP Going Off Duty	Signature of Nurse/LP Coming On Duty	Count Correct?	
				Yes	No

SHIFT COUNT – CONTROLLED DRUGS / MEDS

At each shift change, all controlled drugs / meds must be counted.
Complete *Report of Error in End of Shift Narcotic Count Form* to document any discrepancies.

SHIFT COUNT – CONTROLLED DRUGS / MEDS

Today's Date	Time Of Day	Signature of Nurse/LP Going Off Duty	Signature of Nurse/LP Coming On Duty	Count Correct?	
				Yes	No

At each shift change, all controlled drugs / meds must be counted.
Complete *Report of Error in End of Shift Narcotic Count Form* to document any discrepancies.

SHIFT COUNT – CONTROLLED DRUGS / MEDS

Today's Date	Time Of Day	Signature of Nurse/LP Going Off Duty	Signature of Nurse/LP Coming On Duty	Count Correct?	
				Yes	No

At each shift change, all controlled drugs / meds must be counted.
Complete *Report of Error in End of Shift Narcotic Count Form* to document any discrepancies.

SHIFT COUNT – CONTROLLED DRUGS / MEDS

Today's Date	Time Of Day	Signature of Nurse/LP Going Off Duty	Signature of Nurse/LP Coming On Duty	Count Correct?	
				Yes	No

At each shift change, all controlled drugs / meds must be counted.
Complete *Report of Error in End of Shift Narcotic Count Form* to document any discrepancies.

SHIFT COUNT – CONTROLLED DRUGS / MEDS

Today's Date	Time Of Day	Signature of Nurse/LP Going Off Duty	Signature of Nurse/LP Coming On Duty	Count Correct?	
				Yes	No

At each shift change, all controlled drugs / meds must be counted.
Complete *Report of Error in End of Shift Narcotic Count Form* to document any discrepancies.

SHIFT COUNT – CONTROLLED DRUGS / MEDS

Today's Date	Time Of Day	Signature of Nurse/LP Going Off Duty	Signature of Nurse/LP Coming On Duty	Count Correct?	
				Yes	No

At each shift change, all controlled drugs / meds must be counted.
Complete *Report of Error in End of Shift Narcotic Count Form* to document any discrepancies.

SHIFT COUNT – CONTROLLED DRUGS / MEDS

Today's Date	Time Of Day	Signature of Nurse/LP Going Off Duty	Signature of Nurse/LP Coming On Duty	Count Correct?	
				Yes	No

At each shift change, all controlled drugs / meds must be counted.
Complete *Report of Error in End of Shift Narcotic Count Form* to document any discrepancies.

SHIFT COUNT – CONTROLLED DRUGS / MEDS

Today's Date	Time Of Day	Signature of Nurse/LP Going Off Duty	Signature of Nurse/LP Coming On Duty	Count Correct?	
				Yes	No

At each shift change, all controlled drugs / meds must be counted.
Complete *Report of Error in End of Shift Narcotic Count Form* to document any discrepancies.

SHIFT COUNT – CONTROLLED DRUGS / MEDS

Today's Date	Time Of Day	Signature of Nurse/LP Going Off Duty	Signature of Nurse/LP Coming On Duty	Count Correct?	
				Yes	No

At each shift change, all controlled drugs / meds must be counted.
Complete *Report of Error in End of Shift Narcotic Count Form* to document any discrepancies.

SHIFT COUNT – CONTROLLED DRUGS / MEDS

Today's Date	Time Of Day	Signature of Nurse/LP Going Off Duty	Signature of Nurse/LP Coming On Duty	Count Correct?	
				Yes	No

At each shift change, all controlled drugs / meds must be counted.
Complete *Report of Error in End of Shift Narcotic Count Form* to document any discrepancies.

SHIFT COUNT – CONTROLLED DRUGS / MEDS

Today's Date	Time Of Day	Signature of Nurse/LP Going Off Duty	Signature of Nurse/LP Coming On Duty	Count Correct?	
				Yes	No

At each shift change, all controlled drugs / meds must be counted.
Complete *Report of Error in End of Shift Narcotic Count Form* to document any discrepancies.

SHIFT COUNT – CONTROLLED DRUGS / MEDS

Today's Date	Time Of Day	Signature of Nurse/LP Going Off Duty	Signature of Nurse/LP Coming On Duty	Count Correct?	
				Yes	No

At each shift change, all controlled drugs / meds must be counted.
Complete *Report of Error in End of Shift Narcotic Count Form* to document any discrepancies.

SHIFT COUNT – CONTROLLED DRUGS / MEDS

Today's Date	Time Of Day	Signature of Nurse/LP Going Off Duty	Signature of Nurse/LP Coming On Duty	Count Correct?	
				Yes	No

At each shift change, all controlled drugs / meds must be counted.
Complete *Report of Error in End of Shift Narcotic Count Form* to document any discrepancies.

SHIFT COUNT – CONTROLLED DRUGS / MEDS

Today's Date	Time Of Day	Signature of Nurse/LP Going Off Duty	Signature of Nurse/LP Coming On Duty	Count Correct?	
				Yes	No

At each shift change, all controlled drugs / meds must be counted.
Complete *Report of Error in End of Shift Narcotic Count Form* to document any discrepancies.

SHIFT COUNT – CONTROLLED DRUGS / MEDS

Today's Date	Time Of Day	Signature of Nurse/LP Going Off Duty	Signature of Nurse/LP Coming On Duty	Count Correct?	
				Yes	No

At each shift change, all controlled drugs / meds must be counted.
Complete *Report of Error in End of Shift Narcotic Count Form* to document any discrepancies.

SHIFT COUNT – CONTROLLED DRUGS / MEDS

Today's Date	Time Of Day	Signature of Nurse/LP Going Off Duty	Signature of Nurse/LP Coming On Duty	Count Correct?	
				Yes	No

At each shift change, all controlled drugs / meds must be counted.
Complete *Report of Error in End of Shift Narcotic Count Form* to document any discrepancies.

SHIFT COUNT – CONTROLLED DRUGS / MEDS

Today's Date	Time Of Day	Signature of Nurse/LP Going Off Duty	Signature of Nurse/LP Coming On Duty	Count Correct?	
				Yes	No

At each shift change, all controlled drugs / meds must be counted.
Complete *Report of Error in End of Shift Narcotic Count Form* to document any discrepancies.

SHIFT COUNT – CONTROLLED DRUGS / MEDS

Today's Date	Time Of Day	Signature of Nurse/LP Going Off Duty	Signature of Nurse/LP Coming On Duty	Count Correct?	
				Yes	No

At each shift change, all controlled drugs / meds must be counted.
Complete *Report of Error in End of Shift Narcotic Count Form* to document any discrepancies.

SHIFT COUNT – CONTROLLED DRUGS / MEDS

Today's Date	Time Of Day	Signature of Nurse/LP Going Off Duty	Signature of Nurse/LP Coming On Duty	Count Correct?	
				Yes	No

At each shift change, all controlled drugs / meds must be counted.
Complete *Report of Error in End of Shift Narcotic Count Form* to document any discrepancies.

SHIFT COUNT – CONTROLLED DRUGS / MEDS

Today's Date	Time Of Day	Signature of Nurse/LP Going Off Duty	Signature of Nurse/LP Coming On Duty	Count Correct?	
				Yes	No

At each shift change, all controlled drugs / meds must be counted.
Complete *Report of Error in End of Shift Narcotic Count Form* to document any discrepancies.

SHIFT COUNT – CONTROLLED DRUGS / MEDS

Today's Date	Time Of Day	Signature of Nurse/LP Going Off Duty	Signature of Nurse/LP Coming On Duty	Count Correct?	
				Yes	No

At each shift change, all controlled drugs / meds must be counted.
Complete *Report of Error in End of Shift Narcotic Count Form* to document any discrepancies.

SHIFT COUNT – CONTROLLED DRUGS / MEDS

Today's Date	Time Of Day	Signature of Nurse/LP Going Off Duty	Signature of Nurse/LP Coming On Duty	Count Correct?	
				Yes	No

At each shift change, all controlled drugs / meds must be counted.
Complete *Report of Error in End of Shift Narcotic Count Form* to document any discrepancies.

SHIFT COUNT – CONTROLLED DRUGS / MEDS

Today's Date	Time Of Day	Signature of Nurse/LP Going Off Duty	Signature of Nurse/LP Coming On Duty	Count Correct?	
				Yes	No

At each shift change, all controlled drugs / meds must be counted.
Complete *Report of Error in End of Shift Narcotic Count Form* to document any discrepancies.

SHIFT COUNT – CONTROLLED DRUGS / MEDS

Today's Date	Time Of Day	Signature of Nurse/LP Going Off Duty	Signature of Nurse/LP Coming On Duty	Count Correct?	
				Yes	No

At each shift change, all controlled drugs / meds must be counted.
Complete *Report of Error in End of Shift Narcotic Count Form* to document any discrepancies.

SHIFT COUNT – CONTROLLED DRUGS / MEDS

Today's Date	Time Of Day	Signature of Nurse/LP Going Off Duty	Signature of Nurse/LP Coming On Duty	Count Correct?	
				Yes	No

At each shift change, all controlled drugs / meds must be counted.
Complete *Report of Error in End of Shift Narcotic Count Form* to document any discrepancies.

SHIFT COUNT – CONTROLLED DRUGS / MEDS

Today's Date	Time Of Day	Signature of Nurse/LP Going Off Duty	Signature of Nurse/LP Coming On Duty	Count Correct?	
				Yes	No

At each shift change, all controlled drugs / meds must be counted.
Complete *Report of Error in End of Shift Narcotic Count Form* to document any discrepancies.

SHIFT COUNT – CONTROLLED DRUGS / MEDS

Today's Date	Time Of Day	Signature of Nurse/LP Going Off Duty	Signature of Nurse/LP Coming On Duty	Count Correct?	
				Yes	No

At each shift change, all controlled drugs / meds must be counted.
Complete *Report of Error in End of Shift Narcotic Count Form* to document any discrepancies.

SHIFT COUNT – CONTROLLED DRUGS / MEDS

Today's Date	Time Of Day	Signature of Nurse/LP Going Off Duty	Signature of Nurse/LP Coming On Duty	Count Correct?	
				Yes	No

At each shift change, all controlled drugs / meds must be counted.
Complete *Report of Error in End of Shift Narcotic Count Form* to document any discrepancies.

SHIFT COUNT – CONTROLLED DRUGS / MEDS

Today's Date	Time Of Day	Signature of Nurse/LP Going Off Duty	Signature of Nurse/LP Coming On Duty	Count Correct?	
				Yes	No

At each shift change, all controlled drugs / meds must be counted.
Complete *Report of Error in End of Shift Narcotic Count Form* to document any discrepancies.

SHIFT COUNT – CONTROLLED DRUGS / MEDS

Today's Date	Time Of Day	Signature of Nurse/LP Going Off Duty	Signature of Nurse/LP Coming On Duty	Count Correct?	
				Yes	No

At each shift change, all controlled drugs / meds must be counted.
Complete *Report of Error in End of Shift Narcotic Count Form* to document any discrepancies.

SHIFT COUNT – CONTROLLED DRUGS / MEDS

Today's Date	Time Of Day	Signature of Nurse/LP Going Off Duty	Signature of Nurse/LP Coming On Duty	Count Correct?	
				Yes	No

At each shift change, all controlled drugs / meds must be counted.
Complete *Report of Error in End of Shift Narcotic Count Form* to document any discrepancies.

SHIFT COUNT – CONTROLLED DRUGS / MEDS

Today's Date	Time Of Day	Signature of Nurse/LP Going Off Duty	Signature of Nurse/LP Coming On Duty	Count Correct?	
				Yes	No

At each shift change, all controlled drugs / meds must be counted.
Complete *Report of Error in End of Shift Narcotic Count Form* to document any discrepancies.

SHIFT COUNT – CONTROLLED DRUGS / MEDS

Today's Date	Time Of Day	Signature of Nurse/LP Going Off Duty	Signature of Nurse/LP Coming On Duty	Count Correct?	
				Yes	No

At each shift change, all controlled drugs / meds must be counted.
Complete *Report of Error in End of Shift Narcotic Count Form* to document any discrepancies.

SHIFT COUNT – CONTROLLED DRUGS / MEDS

Today's Date	Time Of Day	Signature of Nurse/LP Going Off Duty	Signature of Nurse/LP Coming On Duty	Count Correct?	
				Yes	No

At each shift change, all controlled drugs / meds must be counted.
Complete *Report of Error in End of Shift Narcotic Count Form* to document any discrepancies.

SHIFT COUNT – CONTROLLED DRUGS / MEDS

Today's Date	Time Of Day	Signature of Nurse/LP Going Off Duty	Signature of Nurse/LP Coming On Duty	Count Correct?	
				Yes	No

At each shift change, all controlled drugs / meds must be counted.
Complete *Report of Error in End of Shift Narcotic Count Form* to document any discrepancies.

CONTROLLED DRUG / MED SUPPLY

Drug / Med Name: _____   Page No: **1**

Drug / Med Given			Present Balance	In From Pharmacy	Patient's Name	Prescriber's Name	Nurse/LP's Signature
Date	Time	Dose					

Two Nurse/LPs must witness and sign the destruction / waste of any controlled drugs / meds.
When folding pages over, the disposition of drugs / meds must be documented appropriately.

CONTROLLED DRUG / MED DISPOSITION

The applicable box below must be completed when this page is folded over.

TRANSFER TO NEW PAGE

New page number transferred to: _____

Remaining quantity being transferred: _____

Date of transfer: _____

Nurse/LP making transfer: _____

TRANSFER TO DIFFERENT LOCATION

New location transferred to: _____

New page number transferred to: _____

Remaining quantity being transferred: _____

Date of transfer: _____

Nurse/LP making transfer: _____

Nurse/LP receiving transfer: _____

SURRENDER TO PERSON

Remaining quantity being surrendered: _____

Nurse/LP making surrender: _____

Person Surrendered To
Printed Name: _____
Signature: _____
- Patient - Responsible Party - Nurse/LP - Administrator - (circle one)

DEPLETION OF DRUG / MED
NONE REMAINING – PAGE FINISHED

Date completed: _____

Nurse/LP completing: _____

CONTROLLED DRUG / MED SUPPLY

Drug / Med Name: Page No: **2**

Drug / Med Given			Present Balance	In From Pharmacy	Patient's Name	Prescriber's Name	Nurse/LP's Signature
Date	Time	Dose					

Two Nurse/LPs must witness and sign the destruction / waste of any controlled drugs / meds.
When folding pages over, the disposition of drugs / meds must be documented appropriately.

CONTROLLED DRUG / MED DISPOSITION

*The applicable box below must be completed
when this page is folded over.*

TRANSFER TO NEW PAGE

New page number transferred to: _____

Remaining quantity being transferred: _____

Date of transfer: _____

Nurse/LP making transfer: _____

TRANSFER TO DIFFERENT LOCATION

New location transferred to: _____

New page number transferred to: _____

Remaining quantity being transferred: _____

Date of transfer: _____

Nurse/LP making transfer: _____

Nurse/LP receiving transfer: _____

SURRENDER TO PERSON

Remaining quantity being surrendered: _____

Nurse/LP making surrender: _____

Person Surrendered To
Printed Name: _____
Signature: _____
- Patient - Responsible Party - Nurse/LP - Administrator -   (circle one)

DEPLETION OF DRUG / MED
NONE REMAINING – PAGE FINISHED

Date completed: _____

Nurse/LP completing: _____

CONTROLLED DRUG / MED SUPPLY

Drug / Med Name: _____ Page No: **3**

Drug / Med Given			Present Balance	In From Pharmacy	Patient's Name	Prescriber's Name	Nurse/LP's Signature
Date	Time	Dose					

Two Nurse/LPs must witness and sign the destruction / waste of any controlled drugs / meds.
When folding pages over, the disposition of drugs / meds must be documented appropriately.

CONTROLLED DRUG / MED DISPOSITION

*The applicable box below must be completed
when this page is folded over.*

TRANSFER TO NEW PAGE

New page number transferred to: _____

Remaining quantity being transferred: _____

Date of transfer: _____

Nurse/LP making transfer: _____

TRANSFER TO DIFFERENT LOCATION

New location transferred to: _____

New page number transferred to: _____

Remaining quantity being transferred: _____

Date of transfer: _____

Nurse/LP making transfer: _____

Nurse/LP receiving transfer: _____

SURRENDER TO PERSON

Remaining quantity being surrendered: _____

Nurse/LP making surrender: _____

Person Surrendered To
Printed Name: _____
Signature: _____
- Patient - Responsible Party - Nurse/LP - Administrator - (circle one)

DEPLETION OF DRUG / MED
NONE REMAINING – PAGE FINISHED

Date completed: _____

Nurse/LP completing: _____

CONTROLLED DRUG / MED SUPPLY

Drug / Med Name: Page No: **4**

Date	Time	Dose	Present Balance	In From Pharmacy	Patient's Name	Prescriber's Name	Nurse/LP's Signature

Column headers grouped under "Drug / Med Given": Date, Time, Dose.

Two Nurse/LPs must witness and sign the destruction / waste of any controlled drugs / meds.
When folding pages over, the disposition of drugs / meds must be documented appropriately.

CONTROLLED DRUG / MED DISPOSITION

The applicable box below must be completed
when this page is folded over.

TRANSFER TO NEW PAGE

New page number transferred to: _____

Remaining quantity being transferred: _____

Date of transfer: _____

Nurse/LP making transfer: _____

TRANSFER TO DIFFERENT LOCATION

New location transferred to: _____

New page number transferred to: _____

Remaining quantity being transferred: _____

Date of transfer: _____

Nurse/LP making transfer: _____

Nurse/LP receiving transfer: _____

SURRENDER TO PERSON

Remaining quantity being surrendered: _____

Nurse/LP making surrender: _____

Person Surrendered To
Printed Name: _____
Signature: _____
- Patient - Responsible Party - Nurse/LP - Administrator - (circle one)

DEPLETION OF DRUG / MED
NONE REMAINING – PAGE FINISHED

Date completed: _____

Nurse/LP completing: _____

CONTROLLED DRUG / MED SUPPLY

Drug / Med Name: Page No: **5**

Date	Time	Dose	Present Balance	In From Pharmacy	Patient's Name	Prescriber's Name	Nurse/LP's Signature

Two Nurse/LPs must witness and sign the destruction / waste of any controlled drugs / meds.
When folding pages over, the disposition of drugs / meds must be documented appropriately.

CONTROLLED DRUG / MED DISPOSITION

The applicable box below must be completed
when this page is folded over.

TRANSFER TO NEW PAGE

New page number transferred to: _____

Remaining quantity being transferred: _____

Date of transfer: _____

Nurse/LP making transfer: _____

TRANSFER TO DIFFERENT LOCATION

New location transferred to: _____

New page number transferred to: _____

Remaining quantity being transferred: _____

Date of transfer: _____

Nurse/LP making transfer: _____

Nurse/LP receiving transfer: _____

SURRENDER TO PERSON

Remaining quantity being surrendered: _____

Nurse/LP making surrender: _____

Person Surrendered To
Printed Name: _____
Signature: _____
- Patient - Responsible Party - Nurse/LP - Administrator - (circle one)

DEPLETION OF DRUG / MED
NONE REMAINING – PAGE FINISHED

Date completed: _____

Nurse/LP completing: _____

CONTROLLED DRUG / MED SUPPLY

Drug / Med Name:

Drug / Med Given			Present Balance	In From Pharmacy	Patient's Name	Prescriber's Name	Nurse/LP's Signature
Date	Time	Dose					

Two Nurse/LPs must witness and sign the destruction / waste of any controlled drugs / meds.
When folding pages over, the disposition of drugs / meds must be documented appropriately.

CONTROLLED DRUG / MED DISPOSITION

*The applicable box below must be completed
when this page is folded over.*

TRANSFER TO NEW PAGE

New page number transferred to: _____

Remaining quantity being transferred: _____

Date of transfer: _____

Nurse/LP making transfer: _____

TRANSFER TO DIFFERENT LOCATION

New location transferred to: _____

New page number transferred to: _____

Remaining quantity being transferred: _____

Date of transfer: _____

Nurse/LP making transfer: _____

Nurse/LP receiving transfer: _____

SURRENDER TO PERSON

Remaining quantity being surrendered: _____

Nurse/LP making surrender: _____

Person Surrendered To
Printed Name: _____
Signature: _____
- Patient - Responsible Party - Nurse/LP - Administrator - (circle one)

DEPLETION OF DRUG / MED
NONE REMAINING – PAGE FINISHED

Date completed: _____

Nurse/LP completing: _____

CONTROLLED DRUG / MED SUPPLY

Drug / Med Name: Page No: **7**

Drug / Med Given			Present Balance	In From Pharmacy	Patient's Name	Prescriber's Name	Nurse/LP's Signature
Date	Time	Dose					

Two Nurse/LPs must witness and sign the destruction / waste of any controlled drugs / meds.
When folding pages over, the disposition of drugs / meds must be documented appropriately.

CONTROLLED DRUG / MED DISPOSITION

*The applicable box below must be completed
when this page is folded over.*

TRANSFER TO NEW PAGE

New page number transferred to: _____

Remaining quantity being transferred: _____

Date of transfer: _____

Nurse/LP making transfer: _____

TRANSFER TO DIFFERENT LOCATION

New location transferred to: _____

New page number transferred to: _____

Remaining quantity being transferred: _____

Date of transfer: _____

Nurse/LP making transfer: _____

Nurse/LP receiving transfer: _____

SURRENDER TO PERSON

Remaining quantity being surrendered: _____

Nurse/LP making surrender: _____

Person Surrendered To
Printed Name: _____
Signature: _____
- Patient - Responsible Party - Nurse/LP - Administrator - (circle one)

DEPLETION OF DRUG / MED
NONE REMAINING – PAGE FINISHED

Date completed: _____

Nurse/LP completing: _____

CONTROLLED DRUG / MED SUPPLY

Drug / Med Name: Page No: **8**

Drug / Med Given			Present Balance	In From Pharmacy	Patient's Name	Prescriber's Name	Nurse/LP's Signature
Date	Time	Dose					

Two Nurse/LPs must witness and sign the destruction / waste of any controlled drugs / meds.
When folding pages over, the disposition of drugs / meds must be documented appropriately.

CONTROLLED DRUG / MED DISPOSITION

*The applicable box below must be completed
when this page is folded over.*

TRANSFER TO NEW PAGE

New page number transferred to: _____

Remaining quantity being transferred: _____

Date of transfer: _____

Nurse/LP making transfer: _____

TRANSFER TO DIFFERENT LOCATION

New location transferred to: _____

New page number transferred to: _____

Remaining quantity being transferred: _____

Date of transfer: _____

Nurse/LP making transfer: _____

Nurse/LP receiving transfer: _____

SURRENDER TO PERSON

Remaining quantity being surrendered: _____

Nurse/LP making surrender: _____

Person Surrendered To
Printed Name: _____
Signature: _____
- Patient - Responsible Party - Nurse/LP - Administrator -   (circle one)

DEPLETION OF DRUG / MED
NONE REMAINING – PAGE FINISHED

Date completed: _____

Nurse/LP completing: _____

CONTROLLED DRUG / MED SUPPLY

Drug / Med Name:

Drug / Med Given			Present Balance	In From Pharmacy	Patient's Name	Prescriber's Name	Nurse/LP's Signature
Date	Time	Dose					

Two Nurse/LPs must witness and sign the destruction / waste of any controlled drugs / meds. When folding pages over, the disposition of drugs / meds must be documented appropriately.

CONTROLLED DRUG / MED DISPOSITION

*The applicable box below must be completed
when this page is folded over.*

TRANSFER TO NEW PAGE

New page number transferred to: _____

Remaining quantity being transferred: _____

Date of transfer: _____

Nurse/LP making transfer: _____

TRANSFER TO DIFFERENT LOCATION

New location transferred to: _____

New page number transferred to: _____

Remaining quantity being transferred: _____

Date of transfer: _____

Nurse/LP making transfer: _____

Nurse/LP receiving transfer: _____

SURRENDER TO PERSON

Remaining quantity being surrendered: _____

Nurse/LP making surrender: _____

Person Surrendered To
Printed Name: _____
Signature: _____
- Patient - Responsible Party - Nurse/LP - Administrator -   (circle one)

DEPLETION OF DRUG / MED
NONE REMAINING – PAGE FINISHED

Date completed: _____

Nurse/LP completing: _____

CONTROLLED DRUG / MED SUPPLY

Drug / Med Name: _____ Page No: **10**

Date	Time	Dose	Present Balance	In From Pharmacy	Patient's Name	Prescriber's Name	Nurse/LP's Signature

The "Drug / Med Given" columns (Date, Time, Dose) are grouped under one header.

Two Nurse/LPs must witness and sign the destruction / waste of any controlled drugs / meds.
When folding pages over, the disposition of drugs / meds must be documented appropriately.

CONTROLLED DRUG / MED DISPOSITION

*The applicable box below must be completed
when this page is folded over.*

TRANSFER TO NEW PAGE

New page number transferred to: _____

Remaining quantity being transferred: _____

Date of transfer: _____

Nurse/LP making transfer: _____

TRANSFER TO DIFFERENT LOCATION

New location transferred to: _____

New page number transferred to: _____

Remaining quantity being transferred: _____

Date of transfer: _____

Nurse/LP making transfer: _____

Nurse/LP receiving transfer: _____

SURRENDER TO PERSON

Remaining quantity being surrendered: _____

Nurse/LP making surrender: _____

Person Surrendered To
Printed Name: _____
Signature: _____
- Patient - Responsible Party - Nurse/LP - Administrator -   (circle one)

DEPLETION OF DRUG / MED
NONE REMAINING – PAGE FINISHED

Date completed: _____

Nurse/LP completing: _____

CONTROLLED DRUG / MED SUPPLY

Drug / Med Name: Page No: **11**

Drug / Med Given			Present Balance	In From Pharmacy	Patient's Name	Prescriber's Name	Nurse/LP's Signature
Date	Time	Dose					

Two Nurse/LPs must witness and sign the destruction / waste of any controlled drugs / meds.
When folding pages over, the disposition of drugs / meds must be documented appropriately.

CONTROLLED DRUG / MED DISPOSITION

*The applicable box below must be completed
when this page is folded over.*

TRANSFER TO NEW PAGE

New page number transferred to: _____

Remaining quantity being transferred: _____

Date of transfer: _____

Nurse/LP making transfer: _____

TRANSFER TO DIFFERENT LOCATION

New location transferred to: _____

New page number transferred to: _____

Remaining quantity being transferred: _____

Date of transfer: _____

Nurse/LP making transfer: _____

Nurse/LP receiving transfer: _____

SURRENDER TO PERSON

Remaining quantity being surrendered: _____

Nurse/LP making surrender: _____

Person Surrendered To
Printed Name: _____
Signature: _____
- Patient - Responsible Party - Nurse/LP - Administrator -   (circle one)

DEPLETION OF DRUG / MED
NONE REMAINING – PAGE FINISHED

Date completed: _____

Nurse/LP completing: _____

CONTROLLED DRUG / MED SUPPLY

Drug / Med Name: _____ Page No: **12**

Drug / Med Given			Present Balance	In From Pharmacy	Patient's Name	Prescriber's Name	Nurse/LP's Signature
Date	Time	Dose					

Two Nurse/LPs must witness and sign the destruction / waste of any controlled drugs / meds.
When folding pages over, the disposition of drugs / meds must be documented appropriately.

CONTROLLED DRUG / MED DISPOSITION

*The applicable box below must be completed
when this page is folded over.*

TRANSFER TO NEW PAGE

New page number transferred to: _____

Remaining quantity being transferred: _____

Date of transfer: _____

Nurse/LP making transfer: _____

TRANSFER TO DIFFERENT LOCATION

New location transferred to: _____

New page number transferred to: _____

Remaining quantity being transferred: _____

Date of transfer: _____

Nurse/LP making transfer: _____

Nurse/LP receiving transfer: _____

SURRENDER TO PERSON

Remaining quantity being surrendered: _____

Nurse/LP making surrender: _____

Person Surrendered To
Printed Name: _____
Signature: _____
- Patient - Responsible Party - Nurse/LP - Administrator - (circle one)

DEPLETION OF DRUG / MED
NONE REMAINING – PAGE FINISHED

Date completed: _____

Nurse/LP completing: _____

CONTROLLED DRUG / MED SUPPLY

| Drug / Med Name: | | | | | | | Page No: | 13 |

Drug / Med Given			Present Balance	In From Pharmacy	Patient's Name	Prescriber's Name	Nurse/LP's Signature
Date	Time	Dose					

Two Nurse/LPs must witness and sign the destruction / waste of any controlled drugs / meds.
When folding pages over, the disposition of drugs / meds must be documented appropriately.

CONTROLLED DRUG / MED DISPOSITION

*The applicable box below must be completed
when this page is folded over.*

TRANSFER TO NEW PAGE

New page number transferred to: _____

Remaining quantity being transferred: _____

Date of transfer: _____

Nurse/LP making transfer: _____

TRANSFER TO DIFFERENT LOCATION

New location transferred to: _____

New page number transferred to: _____

Remaining quantity being transferred: _____

Date of transfer: _____

Nurse/LP making transfer: _____

Nurse/LP receiving transfer: _____

SURRENDER TO PERSON

Remaining quantity being surrendered: _____

Nurse/LP making surrender: _____

Person Surrendered To
Printed Name: _____
Signature: _____
- Patient - Responsible Party - Nurse/LP - Administrator - (circle one)

DEPLETION OF DRUG / MED
NONE REMAINING – PAGE FINISHED

Date completed: _____

Nurse/LP completing: _____

CONTROLLED DRUG / MED SUPPLY

Drug / Med Name: _____

Drug / Med Given			Present Balance	In From Pharmacy	Patient's Name	Prescriber's Name	Nurse/LP's Signature
Date	Time	Dose					

Two Nurse/LPs must witness and sign the destruction / waste of any controlled drugs / meds.
When folding pages over, the disposition of drugs / meds must be documented appropriately.

CONTROLLED DRUG / MED DISPOSITION

*The applicable box below must be completed
when this page is folded over.*

TRANSFER TO NEW PAGE

New page number transferred to: _____

Remaining quantity being transferred: _____

Date of transfer: _____

Nurse/LP making transfer: _____

TRANSFER TO DIFFERENT LOCATION

New location transferred to: _____

New page number transferred to: _____

Remaining quantity being transferred: _____

Date of transfer: _____

Nurse/LP making transfer: _____

Nurse/LP receiving transfer: _____

SURRENDER TO PERSON

Remaining quantity being surrendered: _____

Nurse/LP making surrender: _____

Person Surrendered To
Printed Name: _____
Signature: _____
- Patient - Responsible Party - Nurse/LP - Administrator - (circle one)

DEPLETION OF DRUG / MED
NONE REMAINING – PAGE FINISHED

Date completed: _____

Nurse/LP completing: _____

CONTROLLED DRUG / MED SUPPLY

Drug / Med Name:							Page No:	15

Drug / Med Given			Present Balance	In From Pharmacy	Patient's Name	Prescriber's Name	Nurse/LP's Signature
Date	Time	Dose					

Two Nurse/LPs must witness and sign the destruction / waste of any controlled drugs / meds.
When folding pages over, the disposition of drugs / meds must be documented appropriately.

CONTROLLED DRUG / MED DISPOSITION

The applicable box below must be completed
when this page is folded over.

TRANSFER TO NEW PAGE

New page number transferred to: _____

Remaining quantity being transferred: _____

Date of transfer: _____

Nurse/LP making transfer: _____

TRANSFER TO DIFFERENT LOCATION

New location transferred to: _____

New page number transferred to: _____

Remaining quantity being transferred: _____

Date of transfer: _____

Nurse/LP making transfer: _____

Nurse/LP receiving transfer: _____

SURRENDER TO PERSON

Remaining quantity being surrendered: _____

Nurse/LP making surrender: _____

Person Surrendered To
Printed Name: _____
Signature: _____
- Patient - Responsible Party - Nurse/LP - Administrator - (circle one)

DEPLETION OF DRUG / MED
NONE REMAINING – PAGE FINISHED

Date completed: _____

Nurse/LP completing: _____

CONTROLLED DRUG / MED SUPPLY

Drug / Med Name: ⠀⠀⠀⠀⠀⠀⠀⠀⠀⠀⠀⠀⠀⠀⠀⠀⠀⠀⠀⠀⠀ Page No: **16**

Drug / Med Given			Present Balance	In From Pharmacy	Patient's Name	Prescriber's Name	Nurse/LP's Signature
Date	Time	Dose					

Two Nurse/LPs must witness and sign the destruction / waste of any controlled drugs / meds.
When folding pages over, the disposition of drugs / meds must be documented appropriately.

CONTROLLED DRUG / MED DISPOSITION

*The applicable box below must be completed
when this page is folded over.*

TRANSFER TO NEW PAGE

New page number transferred to: _____

Remaining quantity being transferred: _____

Date of transfer: _____

Nurse/LP making transfer: _____

TRANSFER TO DIFFERENT LOCATION

New location transferred to: _____

New page number transferred to: _____

Remaining quantity being transferred: _____

Date of transfer: _____

Nurse/LP making transfer: _____

Nurse/LP receiving transfer: _____

SURRENDER TO PERSON

Remaining quantity being surrendered: _____

Nurse/LP making surrender: _____

Person Surrendered To
Printed Name: _____
Signature: _____
- Patient - Responsible Party - Nurse/LP - Administrator - (circle one)

DEPLETION OF DRUG / MED
NONE REMAINING – PAGE FINISHED

Date completed: _____

Nurse/LP completing: _____

CONTROLLED DRUG / MED SUPPLY

Drug / Med Name: Page No: **17**

Drug / Med Given			Present Balance	In From Pharmacy	Patient's Name	Prescriber's Name	Nurse/LP's Signature
Date	Time	Dose					

Two Nurse/LPs must witness and sign the destruction / waste of any controlled drugs / meds.
When folding pages over, the disposition of drugs / meds must be documented appropriately.

CONTROLLED DRUG / MED DISPOSITION

*The applicable box below must be completed
when this page is folded over.*

TRANSFER TO NEW PAGE

New page number transferred to: _____

Remaining quantity being transferred: _____

Date of transfer: _____

Nurse/LP making transfer: _____

TRANSFER TO DIFFERENT LOCATION

New location transferred to: _____

New page number transferred to: _____

Remaining quantity being transferred: _____

Date of transfer: _____

Nurse/LP making transfer: _____

Nurse/LP receiving transfer: _____

SURRENDER TO PERSON

Remaining quantity being surrendered: _____

Nurse/LP making surrender: _____

Person Surrendered To
Printed Name: _____
Signature: _____
- Patient - Responsible Party - Nurse/LP - Administrator - (circle one)

DEPLETION OF DRUG / MED
NONE REMAINING – PAGE FINISHED

Date completed: _____

Nurse/LP completing: _____

CONTROLLED DRUG / MED SUPPLY

Drug / Med Name: Page No: **18**

Drug / Med Given			Present Balance	In From Pharmacy	Patient's Name	Prescriber's Name	Nurse/LP's Signature
Date	Time	Dose					

Two Nurse/LPs must witness and sign the destruction / waste of any controlled drugs / meds.
When folding pages over, the disposition of drugs / meds must be documented appropriately.

CONTROLLED DRUG / MED DISPOSITION

The applicable box below must be completed when this page is folded over.

TRANSFER TO NEW PAGE

New page number transferred to: _____

Remaining quantity being transferred: _____

Date of transfer: _____

Nurse/LP making transfer: _____

TRANSFER TO DIFFERENT LOCATION

New location transferred to: _____

New page number transferred to: _____

Remaining quantity being transferred: _____

Date of transfer: _____

Nurse/LP making transfer: _____

Nurse/LP receiving transfer: _____

SURRENDER TO PERSON

Remaining quantity being surrendered: _____

Nurse/LP making surrender: _____

Person Surrendered To
Printed Name: _____
Signature: _____
- Patient - Responsible Party - Nurse/LP - Administrator - (circle one)

DEPLETION OF DRUG / MED
NONE REMAINING – PAGE FINISHED

Date completed: _____

Nurse/LP completing: _____

CONTROLLED DRUG / MED SUPPLY

Drug / Med Name: _____ Page No: **19**

Drug / Med Given			Present Balance	In From Pharmacy	Patient's Name	Prescriber's Name	Nurse/LP's Signature
Date	Time	Dose					

Two Nurse/LPs must witness and sign the destruction / waste of any controlled drugs / meds.
When folding pages over, the disposition of drugs / meds must be documented appropriately.

CONTROLLED DRUG / MED DISPOSITION

*The applicable box below must be completed
when this page is folded over.*

TRANSFER TO NEW PAGE

New page number transferred to: _____

Remaining quantity being transferred: _____

Date of transfer: _____

Nurse/LP making transfer: _____

TRANSFER TO DIFFERENT LOCATION

New location transferred to: _____

New page number transferred to: _____

Remaining quantity being transferred: _____

Date of transfer: _____

Nurse/LP making transfer: _____

Nurse/LP receiving transfer: _____

SURRENDER TO PERSON

Remaining quantity being surrendered: _____

Nurse/LP making surrender: _____

Person Surrendered To
Printed Name: _____
Signature: _____
- Patient - Responsible Party - Nurse/LP - Administrator - (circle one)

DEPLETION OF DRUG / MED
NONE REMAINING – PAGE FINISHED

Date completed: _____

Nurse/LP completing: _____

CONTROLLED DRUG / MED SUPPLY

Drug / Med Name: Page No: **20**

Drug / Med Given			Present Balance	In From Pharmacy	Patient's Name	Prescriber's Name	Nurse/LP's Signature
Date	Time	Dose					

Two Nurse/LPs must witness and sign the destruction / waste of any controlled drugs / meds.
When folding pages over, the disposition of drugs / meds must be documented appropriately.

CONTROLLED DRUG / MED DISPOSITION

*The applicable box below must be completed
when this page is folded over.*

TRANSFER TO NEW PAGE

New page number transferred to: _____

Remaining quantity being transferred: _____

Date of transfer: _____

Nurse/LP making transfer: _____

TRANSFER TO DIFFERENT LOCATION

New location transferred to: _____

New page number transferred to: _____

Remaining quantity being transferred: _____

Date of transfer: _____

Nurse/LP making transfer: _____

Nurse/LP receiving transfer: _____

SURRENDER TO PERSON

Remaining quantity being surrendered: _____

Nurse/LP making surrender: _____

Person Surrendered To
Printed Name: _____
Signature: _____
- Patient - Responsible Party - Nurse/LP - Administrator - (circle one)

DEPLETION OF DRUG / MED
NONE REMAINING – PAGE FINISHED

Date completed: _____

Nurse/LP completing: _____

CONTROLLED DRUG / MED SUPPLY

Drug / Med Name: Page No: **21**

Drug / Med Given			Present Balance	In From Pharmacy	Patient's Name	Prescriber's Name	Nurse/LP's Signature
Date	Time	Dose					

Two Nurse/LPs must witness and sign the destruction / waste of any controlled drugs / meds.
When folding pages over, the disposition of drugs / meds must be documented appropriately.

CONTROLLED DRUG / MED DISPOSITION

The applicable box below must be completed
when this page is folded over.

TRANSFER TO NEW PAGE

New page number transferred to: _____

Remaining quantity being transferred: _____

Date of transfer: _____

Nurse/LP making transfer: _____

TRANSFER TO DIFFERENT LOCATION

New location transferred to: _____

New page number transferred to: _____

Remaining quantity being transferred: _____

Date of transfer: _____

Nurse/LP making transfer: _____

Nurse/LP receiving transfer: _____

SURRENDER TO PERSON

Remaining quantity being surrendered: _____

Nurse/LP making surrender: _____

Person Surrendered To
Printed Name: _____
Signature: _____
- Patient - Responsible Party - Nurse/LP - Administrator - (circle one)

DEPLETION OF DRUG / MED
NONE REMAINING – PAGE FINISHED

Date completed: _____

Nurse/LP completing: _____

CONTROLLED DRUG / MED SUPPLY

Drug / Med Name: Page No: **22**

Drug / Med Given			Present Balance	In From Pharmacy	Patient's Name	Prescriber's Name	Nurse/LP's Signature
Date	Time	Dose					

Two Nurse/LPs must witness and sign the destruction / waste of any controlled drugs / meds.
When folding pages over, the disposition of drugs / meds must be documented appropriately.

CONTROLLED DRUG / MED DISPOSITION

*The applicable box below must be completed
when this page is folded over.*

TRANSFER TO NEW PAGE

New page number transferred to: _____

Remaining quantity being transferred: _____

Date of transfer: _____

Nurse/LP making transfer: _____

TRANSFER TO DIFFERENT LOCATION

New location transferred to: _____

New page number transferred to: _____

Remaining quantity being transferred: _____

Date of transfer: _____

Nurse/LP making transfer: _____

Nurse/LP receiving transfer: _____

SURRENDER TO PERSON

Remaining quantity being surrendered: _____

Nurse/LP making surrender: _____

Person Surrendered To
Printed Name: _____
Signature: _____
- Patient - Responsible Party - Nurse/LP - Administrator - (circle one)

DEPLETION OF DRUG / MED
NONE REMAINING – PAGE FINISHED

Date completed: _____

Nurse/LP completing: _____

CONTROLLED DRUG / MED SUPPLY

Drug / Med Name: _____

Drug / Med Given			Present	In From	Patient's	Prescriber's	Nurse/LP's
Date	Time	Dose	Balance	Pharmacy	Name	Name	Signature

Two Nurse/LPs must witness and sign the destruction / waste of any controlled drugs / meds.
When folding pages over, the disposition of drugs / meds must be documented appropriately.

CONTROLLED DRUG / MED DISPOSITION

*The applicable box below must be completed
when this page is folded over.*

TRANSFER TO NEW PAGE

New page number transferred to: _____

Remaining quantity being transferred: _____

Date of transfer: _____

Nurse/LP making transfer: _____

TRANSFER TO DIFFERENT LOCATION

New location transferred to: _____

New page number transferred to: _____

Remaining quantity being transferred: _____

Date of transfer: _____

Nurse/LP making transfer: _____

Nurse/LP receiving transfer: _____

SURRENDER TO PERSON

Remaining quantity being surrendered: _____

Nurse/LP making surrender: _____

Person Surrendered To
Printed Name: _____
Signature: _____
- Patient - Responsible Party - Nurse/LP - Administrator - (circle one)

DEPLETION OF DRUG / MED
NONE REMAINING – PAGE FINISHED

Date completed: _____

Nurse/LP completing: _____

CONTROLLED DRUG / MED SUPPLY

Drug / Med Name: _____ Page No: **24**

Drug / Med Given			Present Balance	In From Pharmacy	Patient's Name	Prescriber's Name	Nurse/LP's Signature
Date	Time	Dose					

Two Nurse/LPs must witness and sign the destruction / waste of any controlled drugs / meds.
When folding pages over, the disposition of drugs / meds must be documented appropriately.

CONTROLLED DRUG / MED DISPOSITION

*The applicable box below must be completed
when this page is folded over.*

TRANSFER TO NEW PAGE

New page number transferred to: _____

Remaining quantity being transferred: _____

Date of transfer: _____

Nurse/LP making transfer: _____

TRANSFER TO DIFFERENT LOCATION

New location transferred to: _____

New page number transferred to: _____

Remaining quantity being transferred: _____

Date of transfer: _____

Nurse/LP making transfer: _____

Nurse/LP receiving transfer: _____

SURRENDER TO PERSON

Remaining quantity being surrendered: _____

Nurse/LP making surrender: _____

Person Surrendered To
Printed Name: _____
Signature: _____
- Patient - Responsible Party - Nurse/LP - Administrator - (circle one)

DEPLETION OF DRUG / MED
NONE REMAINING – PAGE FINISHED

Date completed: _____

Nurse/LP completing: _____

CONTROLLED DRUG / MED SUPPLY

Drug / Med Name: Page No: **25**

Drug / Med Given			Present Balance	In From Pharmacy	Patient's Name	Prescriber's Name	Nurse/LP's Signature
Date	Time	Dose					

Two Nurse/LPs must witness and sign the destruction / waste of any controlled drugs / meds.
When folding pages over, the disposition of drugs / meds must be documented appropriately.

CONTROLLED DRUG / MED DISPOSITION

*The applicable box below must be completed
when this page is folded over.*

TRANSFER TO NEW PAGE

New page number transferred to: _____

Remaining quantity being transferred: _____

Date of transfer: _____

Nurse/LP making transfer: _____

TRANSFER TO DIFFERENT LOCATION

New location transferred to: _____

New page number transferred to: _____

Remaining quantity being transferred: _____

Date of transfer: _____

Nurse/LP making transfer: _____

Nurse/LP receiving transfer: _____

SURRENDER TO PERSON

Remaining quantity being surrendered: _____

Nurse/LP making surrender: _____

Person Surrendered To
Printed Name: _____
Signature: _____
- Patient - Responsible Party - Nurse/LP - Administrator - (circle one)

DEPLETION OF DRUG / MED
NONE REMAINING – PAGE FINISHED

Date completed: _____

Nurse/LP completing: _____

CONTROLLED DRUG / MED SUPPLY

Drug / Med Name: _____   Page No: **26**

Drug / Med Given			Present Balance	In From Pharmacy	Patient's Name	Prescriber's Name	Nurse/LP's Signature
Date	Time	Dose					

Two Nurse/LPs must witness and sign the destruction / waste of any controlled drugs / meds.
When folding pages over, the disposition of drugs / meds must be documented appropriately.

CONTROLLED DRUG / MED DISPOSITION

The applicable box below must be completed
when this page is folded over.

TRANSFER TO NEW PAGE

New page number transferred to: _____

Remaining quantity being transferred: _____

Date of transfer: _____

Nurse/LP making transfer: _____

TRANSFER TO DIFFERENT LOCATION

New location transferred to: _____

New page number transferred to: _____

Remaining quantity being transferred: _____

Date of transfer: _____

Nurse/LP making transfer: _____

Nurse/LP receiving transfer: _____

SURRENDER TO PERSON

Remaining quantity being surrendered: _____

Nurse/LP making surrender: _____

Person Surrendered To
Printed Name: _____
Signature: _____
- Patient - Responsible Party - Nurse/LP - Administrator - (circle one)

DEPLETION OF DRUG / MED
NONE REMAINING – PAGE FINISHED

Date completed: _____

Nurse/LP completing: _____

CONTROLLED DRUG / MED SUPPLY

Drug / Med Name: Page No: **27**

Drug / Med Given			Present Balance	In From* Pharmacy	Patient's Name	Prescriber's Name	Nurse/LP's Signature
Date	Time	Dose					

Two Nurse/LPs must witness and sign the destruction / waste of any controlled drugs / meds.
When folding pages over, the disposition of drugs / meds must be documented appropriately.

CONTROLLED DRUG / MED DISPOSITION

*The applicable box below must be completed
when this page is folded over.*

TRANSFER TO NEW PAGE

New page number transferred to: _____

Remaining quantity being transferred: _____

Date of transfer: _____

Nurse/LP making transfer: _____

TRANSFER TO DIFFERENT LOCATION

New location transferred to: _____

New page number transferred to: _____

Remaining quantity being transferred: _____

Date of transfer: _____

Nurse/LP making transfer: _____

Nurse/LP receiving transfer: _____

SURRENDER TO PERSON

Remaining quantity being surrendered: _____

Nurse/LP making surrender: _____

Person Surrendered To
Printed Name: _____
Signature: _____
- Patient - Responsible Party - Nurse/LP - Administrator - (circle one)

DEPLETION OF DRUG / MED
NONE REMAINING – PAGE FINISHED

Date completed: _____

Nurse/LP completing: _____

CONTROLLED DRUG / MED SUPPLY

Drug / Med Name: _____ Page No: **28**

Drug / Med Given			Present Balance	In From Pharmacy	Patient's Name	Prescriber's Name	Nurse/LP's Signature
Date	Time	Dose					

Two Nurse/LPs must witness and sign the destruction / waste of any controlled drugs / meds.
When folding pages over, the disposition of drugs / meds must be documented appropriately.

CONTROLLED DRUG / MED DISPOSITION

*The applicable box below must be completed
when this page is folded over.*

TRANSFER TO NEW PAGE

New page number transferred to: _____

Remaining quantity being transferred: _____

Date of transfer: _____

Nurse/LP making transfer: _____

TRANSFER TO DIFFERENT LOCATION

New location transferred to: _____

New page number transferred to: _____

Remaining quantity being transferred: _____

Date of transfer: _____

Nurse/LP making transfer: _____

Nurse/LP receiving transfer: _____

SURRENDER TO PERSON

Remaining quantity being surrendered: _____

Nurse/LP making surrender: _____

Person Surrendered To
Printed Name: _____
Signature: _____
- Patient - Responsible Party - Nurse/LP - Administrator - (circle one)

DEPLETION OF DRUG / MED
NONE REMAINING – PAGE FINISHED

Date completed: _____

Nurse/LP completing: _____

CONTROLLED DRUG / MED SUPPLY

Drug / Med Name:

Drug / Med Given			Present Balance	In From Pharmacy	Patient's Name	Prescriber's Name	Nurse/LP's Signature
Date	Time	Dose					

Two Nurse/LPs must witness and sign the destruction / waste of any controlled drugs / meds.
When folding pages over, the disposition of drugs / meds must be documented appropriately.

CONTROLLED DRUG / MED DISPOSITION

*The applicable box below must be completed
when this page is folded over.*

TRANSFER TO NEW PAGE

New page number transferred to: _____

Remaining quantity being transferred: _____

Date of transfer: _____

Nurse/LP making transfer: _____

TRANSFER TO DIFFERENT LOCATION

New location transferred to: _____

New page number transferred to: _____

Remaining quantity being transferred: _____

Date of transfer: _____

Nurse/LP making transfer: _____

Nurse/LP receiving transfer: _____

SURRENDER TO PERSON

Remaining quantity being surrendered: _____

Nurse/LP making surrender: _____

Person Surrendered To
Printed Name: _____
Signature: _____
- Patient - Responsible Party - Nurse/LP - Administrator -   (circle one)

DEPLETION OF DRUG / MED
NONE REMAINING – PAGE FINISHED

Date completed: _____

Nurse/LP completing: _____

CONTROLLED DRUG / MED SUPPLY

Drug / Med Name: Page No: **30**

Date	Time	Dose	Present Balance	In From Pharmacy	Patient's Name	Prescriber's Name	Nurse/LP's Signature

Two Nurse/LPs must witness and sign the destruction / waste of any controlled drugs / meds.
When folding pages over, the disposition of drugs / meds must be documented appropriately.

CONTROLLED DRUG / MED DISPOSITION

*The applicable box below must be completed
when this page is folded over.*

TRANSFER TO NEW PAGE

New page number transferred to: _____

Remaining quantity being transferred: _____

Date of transfer: _____

Nurse/LP making transfer: _____

TRANSFER TO DIFFERENT LOCATION

New location transferred to: _____

New page number transferred to: _____

Remaining quantity being transferred: _____

Date of transfer: _____

Nurse/LP making transfer: _____

Nurse/LP receiving transfer: _____

SURRENDER TO PERSON

Remaining quantity being surrendered: _____

Nurse/LP making surrender: _____

Person Surrendered To
Printed Name: _____
Signature: _____
- Patient - Responsible Party - Nurse/LP - Administrator - (circle one)

DEPLETION OF DRUG / MED
NONE REMAINING – PAGE FINISHED

Date completed: _____

Nurse/LP completing: _____

CONTROLLED DRUG / MED SUPPLY

Drug / Med Name: Page No: **31**

Drug / Med Given			Present Balance	In From Pharmacy	Patient's Name	Prescriber's Name	Nurse/LP's Signature
Date	Time	Dose					

Two Nurse/LPs must witness and sign the destruction / waste of any controlled drugs / meds.
When folding pages over, the disposition of drugs / meds must be documented appropriately.

CONTROLLED DRUG / MED DISPOSITION

The applicable box below must be completed
when this page is folded over.

TRANSFER TO NEW PAGE

New page number transferred to: _____

Remaining quantity being transferred: _____

Date of transfer: _____

Nurse/LP making transfer: _____

TRANSFER TO DIFFERENT LOCATION

New location transferred to: _____

New page number transferred to: _____

Remaining quantity being transferred: _____

Date of transfer: _____

Nurse/LP making transfer: _____

Nurse/LP receiving transfer: _____

SURRENDER TO PERSON

Remaining quantity being surrendered: _____

Nurse/LP making surrender: _____

Person Surrendered To
Printed Name: _____
Signature: _____
- Patient - Responsible Party - Nurse/LP - Administrator - (circle one)

DEPLETION OF DRUG / MED
NONE REMAINING – PAGE FINISHED

Date completed: _____

Nurse/LP completing: _____

CONTROLLED DRUG / MED SUPPLY

Drug / Med Name: Page No: **32**

Drug / Med Given			Present Balance	In From Pharmacy	Patient's Name	Prescriber's Name	Nurse/LP's Signature
Date	Time	Dose					

Two Nurse/LPs must witness and sign the destruction / waste of any controlled drugs / meds.
When folding pages over, the disposition of drugs / meds must be documented appropriately.

CONTROLLED DRUG / MED DISPOSITION

The applicable box below must be completed
when this page is folded over.

TRANSFER TO NEW PAGE

New page number transferred to: _____

Remaining quantity being transferred: _____

Date of transfer: _____

Nurse/LP making transfer: _____

TRANSFER TO DIFFERENT LOCATION

New location transferred to: _____

New page number transferred to: _____

Remaining quantity being transferred: _____

Date of transfer: _____

Nurse/LP making transfer: _____

Nurse/LP receiving transfer: _____

SURRENDER TO PERSON

Remaining quantity being surrendered: _____

Nurse/LP making surrender: _____

Person Surrendered To
Printed Name: _____
Signature: _____
- Patient - Responsible Party - Nurse/LP - Administrator - (circle one)

DEPLETION OF DRUG / MED
NONE REMAINING – PAGE FINISHED

Date completed: _____

Nurse/LP completing: _____

CONTROLLED DRUG / MED SUPPLY

Drug / Med Name:

Drug / Med Given			Present Balance	In From Pharmacy	Patient's Name	Prescriber's Name	Nurse/LP's Signature
Date	Time	Dose					

Two Nurse/LPs must witness and sign the destruction / waste of any controlled drugs / meds.
When folding pages over, the disposition of drugs / meds must be documented appropriately.

CONTROLLED DRUG / MED DISPOSITION

The applicable box below must be completed
when this page is folded over.

TRANSFER TO NEW PAGE

New page number transferred to: _____

Remaining quantity being transferred: _____

Date of transfer: _____

Nurse/LP making transfer: _____

TRANSFER TO DIFFERENT LOCATION

New location transferred to: _____

New page number transferred to: _____

Remaining quantity being transferred: _____

Date of transfer: _____

Nurse/LP making transfer: _____

Nurse/LP receiving transfer: _____

SURRENDER TO PERSON

Remaining quantity being surrendered: _____

Nurse/LP making surrender: _____

Person Surrendered To
Printed Name: _____
Signature: _____
- Patient - Responsible Party - Nurse/LP - Administrator -   (circle one)

DEPLETION OF DRUG / MED
NONE REMAINING – PAGE FINISHED

Date completed: _____

Nurse/LP completing: _____

CONTROLLED DRUG / MED SUPPLY

Drug / Med Name: Page No: **34**

Drug / Med Given			Present Balance	In From Pharmacy	Patient's Name	Prescriber's Name	Nurse/LP's Signature
Date	Time	Dose					

Two Nurse/LPs must witness and sign the destruction / waste of any controlled drugs / meds.
When folding pages over, the disposition of drugs / meds must be documented appropriately.

CONTROLLED DRUG / MED DISPOSITION

The applicable box below must be completed
when this page is folded over.

TRANSFER TO NEW PAGE

New page number transferred to: _____

Remaining quantity being transferred: _____

Date of transfer: _____

Nurse/LP making transfer: _____

TRANSFER TO DIFFERENT LOCATION

New location transferred to: _____

New page number transferred to: _____

Remaining quantity being transferred: _____

Date of transfer: _____

Nurse/LP making transfer: _____

Nurse/LP receiving transfer: _____

SURRENDER TO PERSON

Remaining quantity being surrendered: _____

Nurse/LP making surrender: _____

Person Surrendered To
Printed Name: _____
Signature: _____
- Patient - Responsible Party - Nurse/LP - Administrator - (circle one)

DEPLETION OF DRUG / MED
NONE REMAINING – PAGE FINISHED

Date completed: _____

Nurse/LP completing: _____

CONTROLLED DRUG / MED SUPPLY

Drug / Med Name: Page No: **35**

Drug / Med Given			Present Balance	In From Pharmacy	Patient's Name	Prescriber's Name	Nurse/LP's Signature
Date	Time	Dose					

Two Nurse/LPs must witness and sign the destruction / waste of any controlled drugs / meds.
When folding pages over, the disposition of drugs / meds must be documented appropriately.

CONTROLLED DRUG / MED DISPOSITION

The applicable box below must be completed
when this page is folded over.

TRANSFER TO NEW PAGE

New page number transferred to: _____

Remaining quantity being transferred: _____

Date of transfer: _____

Nurse/LP making transfer: _____

TRANSFER TO DIFFERENT LOCATION

New location transferred to: _____

New page number transferred to: _____

Remaining quantity being transferred: _____

Date of transfer: _____

Nurse/LP making transfer: _____

Nurse/LP receiving transfer: _____

SURRENDER TO PERSON

Remaining quantity being surrendered: _____

Nurse/LP making surrender: _____

Person Surrendered To
Printed Name: _____
Signature: _____
- Patient - Responsible Party - Nurse/LP - Administrator - (circle one)

DEPLETION OF DRUG / MED
NONE REMAINING – PAGE FINISHED

Date completed: _____

Nurse/LP completing: _____

CONTROLLED DRUG / MED SUPPLY

Drug / Med Name: Page No: **36**

Date	Time	Dose	Present Balance	In From Pharmacy	Patient's Name	Prescriber's Name	Nurse/LP's Signature

Two Nurse/LPs must witness and sign the destruction / waste of any controlled drugs / meds.
When folding pages over, the disposition of drugs / meds must be documented appropriately.

CONTROLLED DRUG / MED DISPOSITION

The applicable box below must be completed
when this page is folded over.

TRANSFER TO NEW PAGE

New page number transferred to: _____

Remaining quantity being transferred: _____

Date of transfer: _____

Nurse/LP making transfer: _____

TRANSFER TO DIFFERENT LOCATION

New location transferred to: _____

New page number transferred to: _____

Remaining quantity being transferred: _____

Date of transfer: _____

Nurse/LP making transfer: _____

Nurse/LP receiving transfer: _____

SURRENDER TO PERSON

Remaining quantity being surrendered: _____

Nurse/LP making surrender: _____

Person Surrendered To
Printed Name: _____
Signature: _____
- Patient - Responsible Party - Nurse/LP - Administrator - (circle one)

DEPLETION OF DRUG / MED
NONE REMAINING – PAGE FINISHED

Date completed: _____

Nurse/LP completing: _____

CONTROLLED DRUG / MED SUPPLY

Drug / Med Name: _____ Page No: **37**

Drug / Med Given			Present Balance	In From Pharmacy	Patient's Name	Prescriber's Name	Nurse/LP's Signature
Date	Time	Dose					

Two Nurse/LPs must witness and sign the destruction / waste of any controlled drugs / meds.
When folding pages over, the disposition of drugs / meds must be documented appropriately.

CONTROLLED DRUG / MED DISPOSITION

*The applicable box below must be completed
when this page is folded over.*

TRANSFER TO NEW PAGE

New page number transferred to: _____

Remaining quantity being transferred: _____

Date of transfer: _____

Nurse/LP making transfer: _____

TRANSFER TO DIFFERENT LOCATION

New location transferred to: _____

New page number transferred to: _____

Remaining quantity being transferred: _____

Date of transfer: _____

Nurse/LP making transfer: _____

Nurse/LP receiving transfer: _____

SURRENDER TO PERSON

Remaining quantity being surrendered: _____

Nurse/LP making surrender: _____

Person Surrendered To
Printed Name: _____
Signature: _____
- Patient - Responsible Party - Nurse/LP - Administrator -   (circle one)

DEPLETION OF DRUG / MED
NONE REMAINING – PAGE FINISHED

Date completed: _____

Nurse/LP completing: _____

CONTROLLED DRUG / MED SUPPLY

Drug / Med Name: Page No: **38**

Drug / Med Given			Present Balance	In From Pharmacy	Patient's Name	Prescriber's Name	Nurse/LP's Signature
Date	Time	Dose					

Two Nurse/LPs must witness and sign the destruction / waste of any controlled drugs / meds.
When folding pages over, the disposition of drugs / meds must be documented appropriately.

CONTROLLED DRUG / MED DISPOSITION

The applicable box below must be completed when this page is folded over.

TRANSFER TO NEW PAGE

New page number transferred to: _____

Remaining quantity being transferred: _____

Date of transfer: _____

Nurse/LP making transfer: _____

TRANSFER TO DIFFERENT LOCATION

New location transferred to: _____

New page number transferred to: _____

Remaining quantity being transferred: _____

Date of transfer: _____

Nurse/LP making transfer: _____

Nurse/LP receiving transfer: _____

SURRENDER TO PERSON

Remaining quantity being surrendered: _____

Nurse/LP making surrender: _____

Person Surrendered To
Printed Name: _____
Signature: _____
- Patient - Responsible Party - Nurse/LP - Administrator - (circle one)

DEPLETION OF DRUG / MED
NONE REMAINING – PAGE FINISHED

Date completed: _____

Nurse/LP completing: _____

CONTROLLED DRUG / MED SUPPLY

Drug / Med Name: _____   Page No: **39**

Drug / Med Given			Present Balance	In From Pharmacy	Patient's Name	Prescriber's Name	Nurse/LP's Signature
Date	Time	Dose					

Two Nurse/LPs must witness and sign the destruction / waste of any controlled drugs / meds.
When folding pages over, the disposition of drugs / meds must be documented appropriately.

CONTROLLED DRUG / MED DISPOSITION

The applicable box below must be completed when this page is folded over.

TRANSFER TO NEW PAGE

New page number transferred to: _____

Remaining quantity being transferred: _____

Date of transfer: _____

Nurse/LP making transfer: _____

TRANSFER TO DIFFERENT LOCATION

New location transferred to: _____

New page number transferred to: _____

Remaining quantity being transferred: _____

Date of transfer: _____

Nurse/LP making transfer: _____

Nurse/LP receiving transfer: _____

SURRENDER TO PERSON

Remaining quantity being surrendered: _____

Nurse/LP making surrender: _____

Person Surrendered To
Printed Name: _____
Signature: _____
- Patient - Responsible Party - Nurse/LP - Administrator - (circle one)

DEPLETION OF DRUG / MED
NONE REMAINING – PAGE FINISHED

Date completed: _____

Nurse/LP completing: _____

CONTROLLED DRUG / MED SUPPLY

Drug / Med Name: _____   Page No: **40**

Drug / Med Given			Present Balance	In From Pharmacy	Patient's Name	Prescriber's Name	Nurse/LP's Signature
Date	Time	Dose					

Two Nurse/LPs must witness and sign the destruction / waste of any controlled drugs / meds.
When folding pages over, the disposition of drugs / meds must be documented appropriately.

CONTROLLED DRUG / MED DISPOSITION

The applicable box below must be completed
when this page is folded over.

TRANSFER TO NEW PAGE

New page number transferred to: _____

Remaining quantity being transferred: _____

Date of transfer: _____

Nurse/LP making transfer: _____

TRANSFER TO DIFFERENT LOCATION

New location transferred to: _____

New page number transferred to: _____

Remaining quantity being transferred: _____

Date of transfer: _____

Nurse/LP making transfer: _____

Nurse/LP receiving transfer: _____

SURRENDER TO PERSON

Remaining quantity being surrendered: _____

Nurse/LP making surrender: _____

Person Surrendered To
Printed Name: _____
Signature: _____
- Patient - Responsible Party - Nurse/LP - Administrator - (circle one)

DEPLETION OF DRUG / MED
NONE REMAINING – PAGE FINISHED

Date completed: _____

Nurse/LP completing: _____

CONTROLLED DRUG / MED SUPPLY

Drug / Med Name: _____   Page No: **41**

Drug / Med Given			Present Balance	In From Pharmacy	Patient's Name	Prescriber's Name	Nurse/LP's Signature
Date	Time	Dose					

Two Nurse/LPs must witness and sign the destruction / waste of any controlled drugs / meds.
When folding pages over, the disposition of drugs / meds must be documented appropriately.

CONTROLLED DRUG / MED DISPOSITION

*The applicable box below must be completed
when this page is folded over.*

TRANSFER TO NEW PAGE

New page number transferred to: _____

Remaining quantity being transferred: _____

Date of transfer: _____

Nurse/LP making transfer: _____

TRANSFER TO DIFFERENT LOCATION

New location transferred to: _____

New page number transferred to: _____

Remaining quantity being transferred: _____

Date of transfer: _____

Nurse/LP making transfer: _____

Nurse/LP receiving transfer: _____

SURRENDER TO PERSON

Remaining quantity being surrendered: _____

Nurse/LP making surrender: _____

Person Surrendered To
Printed Name: _____
Signature: _____
- Patient - Responsible Party - Nurse/LP - Administrator - (circle one)

DEPLETION OF DRUG / MED
NONE REMAINING – PAGE FINISHED

Date completed: _____

Nurse/LP completing: _____

CONTROLLED DRUG / MED SUPPLY

Drug / Med Name: Page No: **42**

Drug / Med Given			Present Balance	In From Pharmacy	Patient's Name	Prescriber's Name	Nurse/LP's Signature
Date	Time	Dose					

Two Nurse/LPs must witness and sign the destruction / waste of any controlled drugs / meds.
When folding pages over, the disposition of drugs / meds must be documented appropriately.

CONTROLLED DRUG / MED DISPOSITION

*The applicable box below must be completed
when this page is folded over.*

TRANSFER TO NEW PAGE

New page number transferred to: _____

Remaining quantity being transferred: _____

Date of transfer: _____

Nurse/LP making transfer: _____

TRANSFER TO DIFFERENT LOCATION

New location transferred to: _____

New page number transferred to: _____

Remaining quantity being transferred: _____

Date of transfer: _____

Nurse/LP making transfer: _____

Nurse/LP receiving transfer: _____

SURRENDER TO PERSON

Remaining quantity being surrendered: _____

Nurse/LP making surrender: _____

Person Surrendered To
Printed Name: _____
Signature: _____
- Patient - Responsible Party - Nurse/LP - Administrator - (circle one)

DEPLETION OF DRUG / MED
NONE REMAINING – PAGE FINISHED

Date completed: _____

Nurse/LP completing: _____

CONTROLLED DRUG / MED SUPPLY

Drug / Med Name: Page No: **43**

Date	Time	Dose	Present Balance	In From Pharmacy	Patient's Name	Prescriber's Name	Nurse/LP's Signature

Column group header: **Drug / Med Given** spans Date, Time, Dose.

Two Nurse/LPs must witness and sign the destruction / waste of any controlled drugs / meds.
When folding pages over, the disposition of drugs / meds must be documented appropriately.

CONTROLLED DRUG / MED DISPOSITION

The applicable box below must be completed
when this page is folded over.

TRANSFER TO NEW PAGE

New page number transferred to: _____

Remaining quantity being transferred: _____

Date of transfer: _____

Nurse/LP making transfer: _____

TRANSFER TO DIFFERENT LOCATION

New location transferred to: _____

New page number transferred to: _____

Remaining quantity being transferred: _____

Date of transfer: _____

Nurse/LP making transfer: _____

Nurse/LP receiving transfer: _____

SURRENDER TO PERSON

Remaining quantity being surrendered: _____

Nurse/LP making surrender: _____

Person Surrendered To
Printed Name: _____
Signature: _____
- Patient - Responsible Party - Nurse/LP - Administrator - (circle one)

DEPLETION OF DRUG / MED
NONE REMAINING – PAGE FINISHED

Date completed: _____

Nurse/LP completing: _____

CONTROLLED DRUG / MED SUPPLY

Drug / Med Name: _____   Page No:

Drug / Med Given			Present Balance	In From Pharmacy	Patient's Name	Prescriber's Name	Nurse/LP's Signature
Date	Time	Dose					

Two Nurse/LPs must witness and sign the destruction / waste of any controlled drugs / meds.
When folding pages over, the disposition of drugs / meds must be documented appropriately.

CONTROLLED DRUG / MED DISPOSITION

The applicable box below must be completed when this page is folded over.

TRANSFER TO NEW PAGE

New page number transferred to: _____

Remaining quantity being transferred: _____

Date of transfer: _____

Nurse/LP making transfer: _____

TRANSFER TO DIFFERENT LOCATION

New location transferred to: _____

New page number transferred to: _____

Remaining quantity being transferred: _____

Date of transfer: _____

Nurse/LP making transfer: _____

Nurse/LP receiving transfer: _____

SURRENDER TO PERSON

Remaining quantity being surrendered: _____

Nurse/LP making surrender: _____

Person Surrendered To
Printed Name: _____
Signature: _____
- Patient - Responsible Party - Nurse/LP - Administrator - (circle one)

DEPLETION OF DRUG / MED
NONE REMAINING – PAGE FINISHED

Date completed: _____

Nurse/LP completing: _____

CONTROLLED DRUG / MED SUPPLY

Drug / Med Name:

Drug / Med Given			Present Balance	In From Pharmacy	Patient's Name	Prescriber's Name	Nurse/LP's Signature
Date	Time	Dose					

Two Nurse/LPs must witness and sign the destruction / waste of any controlled drugs / meds.
When folding pages over, the disposition of drugs / meds must be documented appropriately.

CONTROLLED DRUG / MED DISPOSITION

*The applicable box below must be completed
when this page is folded over.*

TRANSFER TO NEW PAGE

New page number transferred to: _____

Remaining quantity being transferred: _____

Date of transfer: _____

Nurse/LP making transfer: _____

TRANSFER TO DIFFERENT LOCATION

New location transferred to: _____

New page number transferred to: _____

Remaining quantity being transferred: _____

Date of transfer: _____

Nurse/LP making transfer: _____

Nurse/LP receiving transfer: _____

SURRENDER TO PERSON

Remaining quantity being surrendered: _____

Nurse/LP making surrender: _____

Person Surrendered To
Printed Name: _____
Signature: _____
- Patient - Responsible Party - Nurse/LP - Administrator - (circle one)

DEPLETION OF DRUG / MED
NONE REMAINING – PAGE FINISHED

Date completed: _____

Nurse/LP completing: _____

CONTROLLED DRUG / MED SUPPLY

Drug / Med Name: Page No: **46**

Drug / Med Given			Present Balance	In From Pharmacy	Patient's Name	Prescriber's Name	Nurse/LP's Signature
Date	Time	Dose					

Two Nurse/LPs must witness and sign the destruction / waste of any controlled drugs / meds.
When folding pages over, the disposition of drugs / meds must be documented appropriately.

CONTROLLED DRUG / MED DISPOSITION

The applicable box below must be completed
when this page is folded over.

TRANSFER TO NEW PAGE

New page number transferred to: _____

Remaining quantity being transferred: _____

Date of transfer: _____

Nurse/LP making transfer: _____

TRANSFER TO DIFFERENT LOCATION

New location transferred to: _____

New page number transferred to: _____

Remaining quantity being transferred: _____

Date of transfer: _____

Nurse/LP making transfer: _____

Nurse/LP receiving transfer: _____

SURRENDER TO PERSON

Remaining quantity being surrendered: _____

Nurse/LP making surrender: _____

Person Surrendered To
Printed Name: _____
Signature: _____
- Patient - Responsible Party - Nurse/LP - Administrator -   (circle one)

DEPLETION OF DRUG / MED
NONE REMAINING – PAGE FINISHED

Date completed: _____

Nurse/LP completing: _____

CONTROLLED DRUG / MED SUPPLY

Drug / Med Name: _____ Page No: **47**

Drug / Med Given			Present Balance	In From Pharmacy	Patient's Name	Prescriber's Name	Nurse/LP's Signature
Date	Time	Dose					

Two Nurse/LPs must witness and sign the destruction / waste of any controlled drugs / meds.
When folding pages over, the disposition of drugs / meds must be documented appropriately.

CONTROLLED DRUG / MED DISPOSITION

*The applicable box below must be completed
when this page is folded over.*

TRANSFER TO NEW PAGE

New page number transferred to: _____

Remaining quantity being transferred: _____

Date of transfer: _____

Nurse/LP making transfer: _____

TRANSFER TO DIFFERENT LOCATION

New location transferred to: _____

New page number transferred to: _____

Remaining quantity being transferred: _____

Date of transfer: _____

Nurse/LP making transfer: _____

Nurse/LP receiving transfer: _____

SURRENDER TO PERSON

Remaining quantity being surrendered: _____

Nurse/LP making surrender: _____

Person Surrendered To
Printed Name: _____
Signature: _____
- Patient - Responsible Party - Nurse/LP - Administrator -   (circle one)

DEPLETION OF DRUG / MED
NONE REMAINING – PAGE FINISHED

Date completed: _____

Nurse/LP completing: _____

CONTROLLED DRUG / MED SUPPLY

Drug / Med Name: _____ Page No: **48**

Drug / Med Given			Present Balance	In From Pharmacy	Patient's Name	Prescriber's Name	Nurse/LP's Signature
Date	Time	Dose					

Two Nurse/LPs must witness and sign the destruction / waste of any controlled drugs / meds.
When folding pages over, the disposition of drugs / meds must be documented appropriately.

CONTROLLED DRUG / MED DISPOSITION

*The applicable box below must be completed
when this page is folded over.*

TRANSFER TO NEW PAGE

New page number transferred to: _____

Remaining quantity being transferred: _____

Date of transfer: _____

Nurse/LP making transfer: _____

TRANSFER TO DIFFERENT LOCATION

New location transferred to: _____

New page number transferred to: _____

Remaining quantity being transferred: _____

Date of transfer: _____

Nurse/LP making transfer: _____

Nurse/LP receiving transfer: _____

SURRENDER TO PERSON

Remaining quantity being surrendered: _____

Nurse/LP making surrender: _____

Person Surrendered To
Printed Name: _____
Signature: _____
- Patient - Responsible Party - Nurse/LP - Administrator - (circle one)

DEPLETION OF DRUG / MED
NONE REMAINING – PAGE FINISHED

Date completed: _____

Nurse/LP completing: _____

CONTROLLED DRUG / MED SUPPLY

Drug / Med Name:

Date	Time	Dose	Present Balance	In From Pharmacy	Patient's Name	Prescriber's Name	Nurse/LP's Signature

Two Nurse/LPs must witness and sign the destruction / waste of any controlled drugs / meds.
When folding pages over, the disposition of drugs / meds must be documented appropriately.

CONTROLLED DRUG / MED DISPOSITION

*The applicable box below must be completed
when this page is folded over.*

TRANSFER TO NEW PAGE

New page number transferred to: _____

Remaining quantity being transferred: _____

Date of transfer: _____

Nurse/LP making transfer: _____

TRANSFER TO DIFFERENT LOCATION

New location transferred to: _____

New page number transferred to: _____

Remaining quantity being transferred: _____

Date of transfer: _____

Nurse/LP making transfer: _____

Nurse/LP receiving transfer: _____

SURRENDER TO PERSON

Remaining quantity being surrendered: _____

Nurse/LP making surrender: _____

Person Surrendered To
Printed Name: _____
Signature: _____
- Patient - Responsible Party - Nurse/LP - Administrator - (circle one)

DEPLETION OF DRUG / MED
NONE REMAINING – PAGE FINISHED

Date completed: _____

Nurse/LP completing: _____

CONTROLLED DRUG / MED SUPPLY

| Drug / Med Name: | | | | | | | Page No: 50 |

Drug / Med Given			Present Balance	In From Pharmacy	Patient's Name	Prescriber's Name	Nurse/LP's Signature
Date	Time	Dose					

Two Nurse/LPs must witness and sign the destruction / waste of any controlled drugs / meds.
When folding pages over, the disposition of drugs / meds must be documented appropriately.

CONTROLLED DRUG / MED DISPOSITION

*The applicable box below must be completed
when this page is folded over.*

TRANSFER TO NEW PAGE

New page number transferred to: _____

Remaining quantity being transferred: _____

Date of transfer: _____

Nurse/LP making transfer: _____

TRANSFER TO DIFFERENT LOCATION

New location transferred to: _____

New page number transferred to: _____

Remaining quantity being transferred: _____

Date of transfer: _____

Nurse/LP making transfer: _____

Nurse/LP receiving transfer: _____

SURRENDER TO PERSON

Remaining quantity being surrendered: _____

Nurse/LP making surrender: _____

Person Surrendered To
Printed Name: _____
Signature: _____
- Patient - Responsible Party - Nurse/LP - Administrator - (circle one)

DEPLETION OF DRUG / MED
NONE REMAINING – PAGE FINISHED

Date completed: _____

Nurse/LP completing: _____

CONTROLLED DRUG / MED SUPPLY

Drug / Med Name: _____ Page No: **51**

Drug / Med Given			Present Balance	In From Pharmacy	Patient's Name	Prescriber's Name	Nurse/LP's Signature
Date	Time	Dose					

Two Nurse/LPs must witness and sign the destruction / waste of any controlled drugs / meds.
When folding pages over, the disposition of drugs / meds must be documented appropriately.

CONTROLLED DRUG / MED DISPOSITION

*The applicable box below must be completed
when this page is folded over.*

TRANSFER TO NEW PAGE

New page number transferred to: _____

Remaining quantity being transferred: _____

Date of transfer: _____

Nurse/LP making transfer: _____

TRANSFER TO DIFFERENT LOCATION

New location transferred to: _____

New page number transferred to: _____

Remaining quantity being transferred: _____

Date of transfer: _____

Nurse/LP making transfer: _____

Nurse/LP receiving transfer: _____

SURRENDER TO PERSON

Remaining quantity being surrendered: _____

Nurse/LP making surrender: _____

Person Surrendered To
Printed Name: _____
Signature: _____
- Patient - Responsible Party - Nurse/LP - Administrator - (circle one)

DEPLETION OF DRUG / MED
NONE REMAINING – PAGE FINISHED

Date completed: _____

Nurse/LP completing: _____

CONTROLLED DRUG / MED SUPPLY

Drug / Med Name: _____ Page No: **52**

Drug / Med Given			Present Balance	In From Pharmacy	Patient's Name	Prescriber's Name	Nurse/LP's Signature
Date	Time	Dose					

Two Nurse/LPs must witness and sign the destruction / waste of any controlled drugs / meds.
When folding pages over, the disposition of drugs / meds must be documented appropriately.

CONTROLLED DRUG / MED DISPOSITION

*The applicable box below must be completed
when this page is folded over.*

TRANSFER TO NEW PAGE

New page number transferred to: _____

Remaining quantity being transferred: _____

Date of transfer: _____

Nurse/LP making transfer: _____

TRANSFER TO DIFFERENT LOCATION

New location transferred to: _____

New page number transferred to: _____

Remaining quantity being transferred: _____

Date of transfer: _____

Nurse/LP making transfer: _____

Nurse/LP receiving transfer: _____

SURRENDER TO PERSON

Remaining quantity being surrendered: _____

Nurse/LP making surrender: _____

Person Surrendered To
Printed Name: _____
Signature: _____
- Patient - Responsible Party - Nurse/LP - Administrator - (circle one)

DEPLETION OF DRUG / MED
NONE REMAINING – PAGE FINISHED

Date completed: _____

Nurse/LP completing: _____

CONTROLLED DRUG / MED SUPPLY

Drug / Med Name: Page No: **53**

Drug / Med Given			Present Balance	In From Pharmacy	Patient's Name	Prescriber's Name	Nurse/LP's Signature
Date	Time	Dose					

Two Nurse/LPs must witness and sign the destruction / waste of any controlled drugs / meds.
When folding pages over, the disposition of drugs / meds must be documented appropriately.

CONTROLLED DRUG / MED DISPOSITION

*The applicable box below must be completed
when this page is folded over.*

TRANSFER TO NEW PAGE

New page number transferred to: _____

Remaining quantity being transferred: _____

Date of transfer: _____

Nurse/LP making transfer: _____

TRANSFER TO DIFFERENT LOCATION

New location transferred to: _____

New page number transferred to: _____

Remaining quantity being transferred: _____

Date of transfer: _____

Nurse/LP making transfer: _____

Nurse/LP receiving transfer: _____

SURRENDER TO PERSON

Remaining quantity being surrendered: _____

Nurse/LP making surrender: _____

Person Surrendered To
Printed Name: _____
Signature: _____
- Patient - Responsible Party - Nurse/LP - Administrator -   (circle one)

DEPLETION OF DRUG / MED
NONE REMAINING – PAGE FINISHED

Date completed: _____

Nurse/LP completing: _____

CONTROLLED DRUG / MED SUPPLY

Drug / Med Name: Page No: **54**

Drug / Med Given			Present Balance	In From Pharmacy	Patient's Name	Prescriber's Name	Nurse/LP's Signature
Date	Time	Dose					

Two Nurse/LPs must witness and sign the destruction / waste of any controlled drugs / meds.
When folding pages over, the disposition of drugs / meds must be documented appropriately.

CONTROLLED DRUG / MED DISPOSITION

*The applicable box below must be completed
when this page is folded over.*

TRANSFER TO NEW PAGE

New page number transferred to: _____

Remaining quantity being transferred: _____

Date of transfer: _____

Nurse/LP making transfer: _____

TRANSFER TO DIFFERENT LOCATION

New location transferred to: _____

New page number transferred to: _____

Remaining quantity being transferred: _____

Date of transfer: _____

Nurse/LP making transfer: _____

Nurse/LP receiving transfer: _____

SURRENDER TO PERSON

Remaining quantity being surrendered: _____

Nurse/LP making surrender: _____

Person Surrendered To
Printed Name: _____
Signature: _____
- Patient - Responsible Party - Nurse/LP - Administrator - (circle one)

DEPLETION OF DRUG / MED
NONE REMAINING – PAGE FINISHED

Date completed: _____

Nurse/LP completing: _____

CONTROLLED DRUG / MED SUPPLY

Drug / Med Name: _____ Page No: **55**

Drug / Med Given			Present Balance	In From Pharmacy	Patient's Name	Prescriber's Name	Nurse/LP's Signature
Date	Time	Dose					

Two Nurse/LPs must witness and sign the destruction / waste of any controlled drugs / meds.
When folding pages over, the disposition of drugs / meds must be documented appropriately.

CONTROLLED DRUG / MED DISPOSITION

*The applicable box below must be completed
when this page is folded over.*

TRANSFER TO NEW PAGE

New page number transferred to: _____

Remaining quantity being transferred: _____

Date of transfer: _____

Nurse/LP making transfer: _____

TRANSFER TO DIFFERENT LOCATION

New location transferred to: _____

New page number transferred to: _____

Remaining quantity being transferred: _____

Date of transfer: _____

Nurse/LP making transfer: _____

Nurse/LP receiving transfer: _____

SURRENDER TO PERSON

Remaining quantity being surrendered: _____

Nurse/LP making surrender: _____

Person Surrendered To
Printed Name: _____
Signature: _____
- Patient - Responsible Party - Nurse/LP - Administrator - (circle one)

DEPLETION OF DRUG / MED
NONE REMAINING – PAGE FINISHED

Date completed: _____

Nurse/LP completing: _____

CONTROLLED DRUG / MED SUPPLY

Drug / Med Name: Page No: **56**

Drug / Med Given			Present Balance	In From Pharmacy	Patient's Name	Prescriber's Name	Nurse/LP's Signature
Date	Time	Dose					

Two Nurse/LPs must witness and sign the destruction / waste of any controlled drugs / meds.
When folding pages over, the disposition of drugs / meds must be documented appropriately.

CONTROLLED DRUG / MED DISPOSITION

*The applicable box below must be completed
when this page is folded over.*

TRANSFER TO NEW PAGE

New page number transferred to: _____

Remaining quantity being transferred: _____

Date of transfer: _____

Nurse/LP making transfer: _____

TRANSFER TO DIFFERENT LOCATION

New location transferred to: _____

New page number transferred to: _____

Remaining quantity being transferred: _____

Date of transfer: _____

Nurse/LP making transfer: _____

Nurse/LP receiving transfer: _____

SURRENDER TO PERSON

Remaining quantity being surrendered: _____

Nurse/LP making surrender: _____

Person Surrendered To
Printed Name: _____
Signature: _____
- Patient - Responsible Party - Nurse/LP - Administrator - (circle one)

DEPLETION OF DRUG / MED
NONE REMAINING – PAGE FINISHED

Date completed: _____

Nurse/LP completing: _____

CONTROLLED DRUG / MED SUPPLY

Drug / Med Name: Page No: **57**

Drug / Med Given			Present Balance	In From Pharmacy	Patient's Name	Prescriber's Name	Nurse/LP's Signature
Date	Time	Dose					

Two Nurse/LPs must witness and sign the destruction / waste of any controlled drugs / meds.
When folding pages over, the disposition of drugs / meds must be documented appropriately.

CONTROLLED DRUG / MED DISPOSITION

*The applicable box below must be completed
when this page is folded over.*

TRANSFER TO NEW PAGE

New page number transferred to: _____

Remaining quantity being transferred: _____

Date of transfer: _____

Nurse/LP making transfer: _____

TRANSFER TO DIFFERENT LOCATION

New location transferred to: _____

New page number transferred to: _____

Remaining quantity being transferred: _____

Date of transfer: _____

Nurse/LP making transfer: _____

Nurse/LP receiving transfer: _____

SURRENDER TO PERSON

Remaining quantity being surrendered: _____

Nurse/LP making surrender: _____

Person Surrendered To
Printed Name: _____
Signature: _____
- Patient - Responsible Party - Nurse/LP - Administrator - (circle one)

DEPLETION OF DRUG / MED
NONE REMAINING – PAGE FINISHED

Date completed: _____

Nurse/LP completing: _____

CONTROLLED DRUG / MED SUPPLY

Drug / Med Name: _____

Drug / Med Given			Present Balance	In From Pharmacy	Patient's Name	Prescriber's Name	Nurse/LP's Signature
Date	Time	Dose					

Two Nurse/LPs must witness and sign the destruction / waste of any controlled drugs / meds.
When folding pages over, the disposition of drugs / meds must be documented appropriately.

CONTROLLED DRUG / MED DISPOSITION

*The applicable box below must be completed
when this page is folded over.*

TRANSFER TO NEW PAGE

New page number transferred to: _____

Remaining quantity being transferred: _____

Date of transfer: _____

Nurse/LP making transfer: _____

TRANSFER TO DIFFERENT LOCATION

New location transferred to: _____

New page number transferred to: _____

Remaining quantity being transferred: _____

Date of transfer: _____

Nurse/LP making transfer: _____

Nurse/LP receiving transfer: _____

SURRENDER TO PERSON

Remaining quantity being surrendered: _____

Nurse/LP making surrender: _____

Person Surrendered To
Printed Name: _____
Signature: _____
- Patient - Responsible Party - Nurse/LP - Administrator - (circle one)

DEPLETION OF DRUG / MED
NONE REMAINING – PAGE FINISHED

Date completed: _____

Nurse/LP completing: _____

CONTROLLED DRUG / MED SUPPLY

Drug / Med Name: ⬚ Page No: **59**

Drug / Med Given			Present Balance	In From Pharmacy	Patient's Name	Prescriber's Name	Nurse/LP's Signature
Date	Time	Dose					

Two Nurse/LPs must witness and sign the destruction / waste of any controlled drugs / meds.
When folding pages over, the disposition of drugs / meds must be documented appropriately.

CONTROLLED DRUG / MED DISPOSITION

*The applicable box below must be completed
when this page is folded over.*

TRANSFER TO NEW PAGE

New page number transferred to: _____

Remaining quantity being transferred: _____

Date of transfer: _____

Nurse/LP making transfer: _____

TRANSFER TO DIFFERENT LOCATION

New location transferred to: _____

New page number transferred to: _____

Remaining quantity being transferred: _____

Date of transfer: _____

Nurse/LP making transfer: _____

Nurse/LP receiving transfer: _____

SURRENDER TO PERSON

Remaining quantity being surrendered: _____

Nurse/LP making surrender: _____

Person Surrendered To
Printed Name: _____
Signature: _____
- Patient - Responsible Party - Nurse/LP - Administrator - (circle one)

DEPLETION OF DRUG / MED
NONE REMAINING – PAGE FINISHED

Date completed: _____

Nurse/LP completing: _____

CONTROLLED DRUG / MED SUPPLY

Drug / Med Name: _____ Page No: **60**

Drug / Med Given			Present Balance	In From Pharmacy	Patient's Name	Prescriber's Name	Nurse/LP's Signature
Date	Time	Dose					

Two Nurse/LPs must witness and sign the destruction / waste of any controlled drugs / meds.
When folding pages over, the disposition of drugs / meds must be documented appropriately.

CONTROLLED DRUG / MED DISPOSITION

The applicable box below must be completed when this page is folded over.

TRANSFER TO NEW PAGE

New page number transferred to: _____

Remaining quantity being transferred: _____

Date of transfer: _____

Nurse/LP making transfer: _____

TRANSFER TO DIFFERENT LOCATION

New location transferred to: _____

New page number transferred to: _____

Remaining quantity being transferred: _____

Date of transfer: _____

Nurse/LP making transfer: _____

Nurse/LP receiving transfer: _____

SURRENDER TO PERSON

Remaining quantity being surrendered: _____

Nurse/LP making surrender: _____

Person Surrendered To
Printed Name: _____
Signature: _____
- Patient - Responsible Party - Nurse/LP - Administrator - (circle one)

DEPLETION OF DRUG / MED
NONE REMAINING – PAGE FINISHED

Date completed: _____

Nurse/LP completing: _____

CONTROLLED DRUG / MED SUPPLY

Drug / Med Name:

Drug / Med Given			Present Balance	In From Pharmacy	Patient's Name	Prescriber's Name	Nurse/LP's Signature
Date	Time	Dose					

Two Nurse/LPs must witness and sign the destruction / waste of any controlled drugs / meds.
When folding pages over, the disposition of drugs / meds must be documented appropriately.

CONTROLLED DRUG / MED DISPOSITION

The applicable box below must be completed
when this page is folded over.

TRANSFER TO NEW PAGE

New page number transferred to: _____

Remaining quantity being transferred: _____

Date of transfer: _____

Nurse/LP making transfer: _____

TRANSFER TO DIFFERENT LOCATION

New location transferred to: _____

New page number transferred to: _____

Remaining quantity being transferred: _____

Date of transfer: _____

Nurse/LP making transfer: _____

Nurse/LP receiving transfer: _____

SURRENDER TO PERSON

Remaining quantity being surrendered: _____

Nurse/LP making surrender: _____

Person Surrendered To
Printed Name: _____
Signature: _____
- Patient - Responsible Party - Nurse/LP - Administrator - (circle one)

DEPLETION OF DRUG / MED
NONE REMAINING – PAGE FINISHED

Date completed: _____

Nurse/LP completing: _____

CONTROLLED DRUG / MED SUPPLY

Drug / Med Name: Page No: **62**

Drug / Med Given			Present Balance	In From Pharmacy	Patient's Name	Prescriber's Name	Nurse/LP's Signature
Date	Time	Dose					

Two Nurse/LPs must witness and sign the destruction / waste of any controlled drugs / meds.
When folding pages over, the disposition of drugs / meds must be documented appropriately.

CONTROLLED DRUG / MED DISPOSITION

The applicable box below must be completed
when this page is folded over.

TRANSFER TO NEW PAGE

New page number transferred to: _____

Remaining quantity being transferred: _____

Date of transfer: _____

Nurse/LP making transfer: _____

TRANSFER TO DIFFERENT LOCATION

New location transferred to: _____

New page number transferred to: _____

Remaining quantity being transferred: _____

Date of transfer: _____

Nurse/LP making transfer: _____

Nurse/LP receiving transfer: _____

SURRENDER TO PERSON

Remaining quantity being surrendered: _____

Nurse/LP making surrender: _____

Person Surrendered To
Printed Name: _____
Signature: _____
- Patient - Responsible Party - Nurse/LP - Administrator - (circle one)

DEPLETION OF DRUG / MED
NONE REMAINING – PAGE FINISHED

Date completed: _____

Nurse/LP completing: _____

CONTROLLED DRUG / MED SUPPLY

Drug / Med Name: Page No: **63**

Drug / Med Given			Present Balance	In From Pharmacy	Patient's Name	Prescriber's Name	Nurse/LP's Signature
Date	Time	Dose					

Two Nurse/LPs must witness and sign the destruction / waste of any controlled drugs / meds.
When folding pages over, the disposition of drugs / meds must be documented appropriately.

CONTROLLED DRUG / MED DISPOSITION

*The applicable box below must be completed
when this page is folded over.*

TRANSFER TO NEW PAGE

New page number transferred to: _____

Remaining quantity being transferred: _____

Date of transfer: _____

Nurse/LP making transfer: _____

TRANSFER TO DIFFERENT LOCATION

New location transferred to: _____

New page number transferred to: _____

Remaining quantity being transferred: _____

Date of transfer: _____

Nurse/LP making transfer: _____

Nurse/LP receiving transfer: _____

SURRENDER TO PERSON

Remaining quantity being surrendered: _____

Nurse/LP making surrender: _____

Person Surrendered To
Printed Name: _____
Signature: _____
- Patient - Responsible Party - Nurse/LP - Administrator - (circle one)

DEPLETION OF DRUG / MED
NONE REMAINING – PAGE FINISHED

Date completed: _____

Nurse/LP completing: _____

CONTROLLED DRUG / MED SUPPLY

Drug / Med Name: _____ Page No: **64**

Drug / Med Given			Present Balance	In From Pharmacy	Patient's Name	Prescriber's Name	Nurse/LP's Signature
Date	Time	Dose					

Two Nurse/LPs must witness and sign the destruction / waste of any controlled drugs / meds.
When folding pages over, the disposition of drugs / meds must be documented appropriately.

CONTROLLED DRUG / MED DISPOSITION

The applicable box below must be completed
when this page is folded over.

TRANSFER TO NEW PAGE

New page number transferred to: _____

Remaining quantity being transferred: _____

Date of transfer: _____

Nurse/LP making transfer: _____

TRANSFER TO DIFFERENT LOCATION

New location transferred to: _____

New page number transferred to: _____

Remaining quantity being transferred: _____

Date of transfer: _____

Nurse/LP making transfer: _____

Nurse/LP receiving transfer: _____

SURRENDER TO PERSON

Remaining quantity being surrendered: _____

Nurse/LP making surrender: _____

Person Surrendered To
Printed Name: _____
Signature: _____
- Patient - Responsible Party - Nurse/LP - Administrator - (circle one)

DEPLETION OF DRUG / MED
NONE REMAINING – PAGE FINISHED

Date completed: _____

Nurse/LP completing: _____

CONTROLLED DRUG / MED SUPPLY

Drug / Med Name: _____   Page No: **65**

Drug / Med Given			Present Balance	In From Pharmacy	Patient's Name	Prescriber's Name	Nurse/LP's Signature
Date	Time	Dose					

Two Nurse/LPs must witness and sign the destruction / waste of any controlled drugs / meds.
When folding pages over, the disposition of drugs / meds must be documented appropriately.

CONTROLLED DRUG / MED DISPOSITION

The applicable box below must be completed when this page is folded over.

TRANSFER TO NEW PAGE

New page number transferred to: _____

Remaining quantity being transferred: _____

Date of transfer: _____

Nurse/LP making transfer: _____

TRANSFER TO DIFFERENT LOCATION

New location transferred to: _____

New page number transferred to: _____

Remaining quantity being transferred: _____

Date of transfer: _____

Nurse/LP making transfer: _____

Nurse/LP receiving transfer: _____

SURRENDER TO PERSON

Remaining quantity being surrendered: _____

Nurse/LP making surrender: _____

Person Surrendered To
Printed Name: _____
Signature: _____
- Patient - Responsible Party - Nurse/LP - Administrator - (circle one)

DEPLETION OF DRUG / MED
NONE REMAINING – PAGE FINISHED

Date completed: _____

Nurse/LP completing: _____

CONTROLLED DRUG / MED SUPPLY

Drug / Med Name: Page No: **66**

Drug / Med Given			Present Balance	In From Pharmacy	Patient's Name	Prescriber's Name	Nurse/LP's Signature
Date	Time	Dose					

Two Nurse/LPs must witness and sign the destruction / waste of any controlled drugs / meds.
When folding pages over, the disposition of drugs / meds must be documented appropriately.

CONTROLLED DRUG / MED DISPOSITION

*The applicable box below must be completed
when this page is folded over.*

TRANSFER TO NEW PAGE

New page number transferred to: _____

Remaining quantity being transferred: _____

Date of transfer: _____

Nurse/LP making transfer: _____

TRANSFER TO DIFFERENT LOCATION

New location transferred to: _____

New page number transferred to: _____

Remaining quantity being transferred: _____

Date of transfer: _____

Nurse/LP making transfer: _____

Nurse/LP receiving transfer: _____

SURRENDER TO PERSON

Remaining quantity being surrendered: _____

Nurse/LP making surrender: _____

Person Surrendered To
Printed Name: _____
Signature: _____
- Patient - Responsible Party - Nurse/LP - Administrator - (circle one)

DEPLETION OF DRUG / MED
NONE REMAINING – PAGE FINISHED

Date completed: _____

Nurse/LP completing: _____

CONTROLLED DRUG / MED SUPPLY

Drug / Med Name: _____   Page No: **67**

Drug / Med Given			Present Balance	In From Pharmacy	Patient's Name	Prescriber's Name	Nurse/LP's Signature
Date	Time	Dose					

Two Nurse/LPs must witness and sign the destruction / waste of any controlled drugs / meds.
When folding pages over, the disposition of drugs / meds must be documented appropriately.

CONTROLLED DRUG / MED DISPOSITION

The applicable box below must be completed when this page is folded over.

TRANSFER TO NEW PAGE

New page number transferred to: _____

Remaining quantity being transferred: _____

Date of transfer: _____

Nurse/LP making transfer: _____

TRANSFER TO DIFFERENT LOCATION

New location transferred to: _____

New page number transferred to: _____

Remaining quantity being transferred: _____

Date of transfer: _____

Nurse/LP making transfer: _____

Nurse/LP receiving transfer: _____

SURRENDER TO PERSON

Remaining quantity being surrendered: _____

Nurse/LP making surrender: _____

Person Surrendered To
Printed Name: _____
Signature: _____
- Patient - Responsible Party - Nurse/LP - Administrator - (circle one)

DEPLETION OF DRUG / MED
NONE REMAINING – PAGE FINISHED

Date completed: _____

Nurse/LP completing: _____

CONTROLLED DRUG / MED SUPPLY

Drug / Med Name: Page No: **68**

Drug / Med Given			Present Balance	In From Pharmacy	Patient's Name	Prescriber's Name	Nurse/LP's Signature
Date	Time	Dose					

Two Nurse/LPs must witness and sign the destruction / waste of any controlled drugs / meds.
When folding pages over, the disposition of drugs / meds must be documented appropriately.

CONTROLLED DRUG / MED DISPOSITION

*The applicable box below must be completed
when this page is folded over.*

TRANSFER TO NEW PAGE

New page number transferred to: _____

Remaining quantity being transferred: _____

Date of transfer: _____

Nurse/LP making transfer: _____

TRANSFER TO DIFFERENT LOCATION

New location transferred to: _____

New page number transferred to: _____

Remaining quantity being transferred: _____

Date of transfer: _____

Nurse/LP making transfer: _____

Nurse/LP receiving transfer: _____

SURRENDER TO PERSON

Remaining quantity being surrendered: _____

Nurse/LP making surrender: _____

Person Surrendered To
Printed Name: _____
Signature: _____
- Patient - Responsible Party - Nurse/LP - Administrator - (circle one)

DEPLETION OF DRUG / MED
NONE REMAINING – PAGE FINISHED

Date completed: _____

Nurse/LP completing: _____

CONTROLLED DRUG / MED SUPPLY

Drug / Med Name:

Drug / Med Given			Present Balance	In From Pharmacy	Patient's Name	Prescriber's Name	Nurse/LP's Signature
Date	Time	Dose					

Two Nurse/LPs must witness and sign the destruction / waste of any controlled drugs / meds.
When folding pages over, the disposition of drugs / meds must be documented appropriately.

CONTROLLED DRUG / MED DISPOSITION

*The applicable box below must be completed
when this page is folded over.*

TRANSFER TO NEW PAGE

New page number transferred to: _____

Remaining quantity being transferred: _____

Date of transfer: _____

Nurse/LP making transfer: _____

TRANSFER TO DIFFERENT LOCATION

New location transferred to: _____

New page number transferred to: _____

Remaining quantity being transferred: _____

Date of transfer: _____

Nurse/LP making transfer: _____

Nurse/LP receiving transfer: _____

SURRENDER TO PERSON

Remaining quantity being surrendered: _____

Nurse/LP making surrender: _____

Person Surrendered To
Printed Name: _____
Signature: _____
- Patient - Responsible Party - Nurse/LP - Administrator - (circle one)

DEPLETION OF DRUG / MED
NONE REMAINING – PAGE FINISHED

Date completed: _____

Nurse/LP completing: _____

CONTROLLED DRUG / MED SUPPLY

Drug / Med Name: _____ Page No: **70**

Drug / Med Given			Present Balance	In From Pharmacy	Patient's Name	Prescriber's Name	Nurse/LP's Signature
Date	Time	Dose					

Two Nurse/LPs must witness and sign the destruction / waste of any controlled drugs / meds.
When folding pages over, the disposition of drugs / meds must be documented appropriately.

CONTROLLED DRUG / MED DISPOSITION

The applicable box below must be completed
when this page is folded over.

TRANSFER TO NEW PAGE

New page number transferred to: _____

Remaining quantity being transferred: _____

Date of transfer: _____

Nurse/LP making transfer: _____

TRANSFER TO DIFFERENT LOCATION

New location transferred to: _____

New page number transferred to: _____

Remaining quantity being transferred: _____

Date of transfer: _____

Nurse/LP making transfer: _____

Nurse/LP receiving transfer: _____

SURRENDER TO PERSON

Remaining quantity being surrendered: _____

Nurse/LP making surrender: _____

Person Surrendered To
Printed Name: _____
Signature: _____
- Patient - Responsible Party - Nurse/LP - Administrator - (circle one)

DEPLETION OF DRUG / MED
NONE REMAINING – PAGE FINISHED

Date completed: _____

Nurse/LP completing: _____

CONTROLLED DRUG / MED SUPPLY

Drug / Med Name: _____ Page No: **71**

Drug / Med Given			Present Balance	In From Pharmacy	Patient's Name	Prescriber's Name	Nurse/LP's Signature
Date	Time	Dose					

Two Nurse/LPs must witness and sign the destruction / waste of any controlled drugs / meds.
When folding pages over, the disposition of drugs / meds must be documented appropriately.

CONTROLLED DRUG / MED DISPOSITION

*The applicable box below must be completed
when this page is folded over.*

TRANSFER TO NEW PAGE

New page number transferred to: _____

Remaining quantity being transferred: _____

Date of transfer: _____

Nurse/LP making transfer: _____

TRANSFER TO DIFFERENT LOCATION

New location transferred to: _____

New page number transferred to: _____

Remaining quantity being transferred: _____

Date of transfer: _____

Nurse/LP making transfer: _____

Nurse/LP receiving transfer: _____

SURRENDER TO PERSON

Remaining quantity being surrendered: _____

Nurse/LP making surrender: _____

Person Surrendered To
Printed Name: _____
Signature: _____
- Patient - Responsible Party - Nurse/LP - Administrator -   (circle one)

DEPLETION OF DRUG / MED
NONE REMAINING – PAGE FINISHED

Date completed: _____

Nurse/LP completing: _____

CONTROLLED DRUG / MED SUPPLY

Drug / Med Name:

Drug / Med Given			Present Balance	In From Pharmacy	Patient's Name	Prescriber's Name	Nurse/LP's Signature
Date	Time	Dose					

Two Nurse/LPs must witness and sign the destruction / waste of any controlled drugs / meds.
When folding pages over, the disposition of drugs / meds must be documented appropriately.

CONTROLLED DRUG / MED DISPOSITION

*The applicable box below must be completed
when this page is folded over.*

TRANSFER TO NEW PAGE

New page number transferred to: _____

Remaining quantity being transferred: _____

Date of transfer: _____

Nurse/LP making transfer: _____

TRANSFER TO DIFFERENT LOCATION

New location transferred to: _____

New page number transferred to: _____

Remaining quantity being transferred: _____

Date of transfer: _____

Nurse/LP making transfer: _____

Nurse/LP receiving transfer: _____

SURRENDER TO PERSON

Remaining quantity being surrendered: _____

Nurse/LP making surrender: _____

Person Surrendered To
Printed Name: _____
Signature: _____
- Patient - Responsible Party - Nurse/LP - Administrator - (circle one)

DEPLETION OF DRUG / MED
NONE REMAINING – PAGE FINISHED

Date completed: _____

Nurse/LP completing: _____

CONTROLLED DRUG / MED SUPPLY

Drug / Med Name: Page No: **73**

Drug / Med Given			Present Balance	In From Pharmacy	Patient's Name	Prescriber's Name	Nurse/LP's Signature
Date	Time	Dose					

Two Nurse/LPs must witness and sign the destruction / waste of any controlled drugs / meds.
When folding pages over, the disposition of drugs / meds must be documented appropriately.

CONTROLLED DRUG / MED DISPOSITION

*The applicable box below must be completed
when this page is folded over.*

TRANSFER TO NEW PAGE

New page number transferred to: _____

Remaining quantity being transferred: _____

Date of transfer: _____

Nurse/LP making transfer: _____

TRANSFER TO DIFFERENT LOCATION

New location transferred to: _____

New page number transferred to: _____

Remaining quantity being transferred: _____

Date of transfer: _____

Nurse/LP making transfer: _____

Nurse/LP receiving transfer: _____

SURRENDER TO PERSON

Remaining quantity being surrendered: _____

Nurse/LP making surrender: _____

Person Surrendered To
Printed Name: _____
Signature: _____
- Patient - Responsible Party - Nurse/LP - Administrator - (circle one)

DEPLETION OF DRUG / MED
NONE REMAINING – PAGE FINISHED

Date completed: _____

Nurse/LP completing: _____

CONTROLLED DRUG / MED SUPPLY

Drug / Med Name: _____   Page No: **74**

Drug / Med Given			Present Balance	In From Pharmacy	Patient's Name	Prescriber's Name	Nurse/LP's Signature
Date	Time	Dose					

Two Nurse/LPs must witness and sign the destruction / waste of any controlled drugs / meds.
When folding pages over, the disposition of drugs / meds must be documented appropriately.

CONTROLLED DRUG / MED DISPOSITION

*The applicable box below must be completed
when this page is folded over.*

TRANSFER TO NEW PAGE

New page number transferred to: _____

Remaining quantity being transferred: _____

Date of transfer: _____

Nurse/LP making transfer: _____

TRANSFER TO DIFFERENT LOCATION

New location transferred to: _____

New page number transferred to: _____

Remaining quantity being transferred: _____

Date of transfer: _____

Nurse/LP making transfer: _____

Nurse/LP receiving transfer: _____

SURRENDER TO PERSON

Remaining quantity being surrendered: _____

Nurse/LP making surrender: _____

Person Surrendered To
Printed Name: _____
Signature: _____
- Patient - Responsible Party - Nurse/LP - Administrator -   (circle one)

DEPLETION OF DRUG / MED
NONE REMAINING – PAGE FINISHED

Date completed: _____

Nurse/LP completing: _____

CONTROLLED DRUG / MED SUPPLY

Drug / Med Name: Page No: **75**

Drug / Med Given			Present Balance	In From Pharmacy	Patient's Name	Prescriber's Name	Nurse/LP's Signature
Date	Time	Dose					

Two Nurse/LPs must witness and sign the destruction / waste of any controlled drugs / meds.
When folding pages over, the disposition of drugs / meds must be documented appropriately.

CONTROLLED DRUG / MED DISPOSITION

*The applicable box below must be completed
when this page is folded over.*

TRANSFER TO NEW PAGE

New page number transferred to: _____

Remaining quantity being transferred: _____

Date of transfer: _____

Nurse/LP making transfer: _____

TRANSFER TO DIFFERENT LOCATION

New location transferred to: _____

New page number transferred to: _____

Remaining quantity being transferred: _____

Date of transfer: _____

Nurse/LP making transfer: _____

Nurse/LP receiving transfer: _____

SURRENDER TO PERSON

Remaining quantity being surrendered: _____

Nurse/LP making surrender: _____

Person Surrendered To
Printed Name: _____
Signature: _____
- Patient - Responsible Party - Nurse/LP - Administrator - (circle one)

DEPLETION OF DRUG / MED
NONE REMAINING – PAGE FINISHED

Date completed: _____

Nurse/LP completing: _____

CONTROLLED DRUG / MED SUPPLY

Drug / Med Name: _____   Page No: **76**

Drug / Med Given			Present Balance	In From Pharmacy	Patient's Name	Prescriber's Name	Nurse/LP's Signature
Date	Time	Dose					

Two Nurse/LPs must witness and sign the destruction / waste of any controlled drugs / meds.
When folding pages over, the disposition of drugs / meds must be documented appropriately.

CONTROLLED DRUG / MED DISPOSITION

*The applicable box below must be completed
when this page is folded over.*

TRANSFER TO NEW PAGE

New page number transferred to: _____

Remaining quantity being transferred: _____

Date of transfer: _____

Nurse/LP making transfer: _____

TRANSFER TO DIFFERENT LOCATION

New location transferred to: _____

New page number transferred to: _____

Remaining quantity being transferred: _____

Date of transfer: _____

Nurse/LP making transfer: _____

Nurse/LP receiving transfer: _____

SURRENDER TO PERSON

Remaining quantity being surrendered: _____

Nurse/LP making surrender: _____

Person Surrendered To
Printed Name: _____
Signature: _____
- Patient - Responsible Party - Nurse/LP - Administrator -   (circle one)

DEPLETION OF DRUG / MED
NONE REMAINING – PAGE FINISHED

Date completed: _____

Nurse/LP completing: _____

CONTROLLED DRUG / MED SUPPLY

Drug / Med Name: _____   Page No: **77**

Drug / Med Given			Present Balance	In From Pharmacy	Patient's Name	Prescriber's Name	Nurse/LP's Signature
Date	Time	Dose					

Two Nurse/LPs must witness and sign the destruction / waste of any controlled drugs / meds.
When folding pages over, the disposition of drugs / meds must be documented appropriately.

CONTROLLED DRUG / MED DISPOSITION

*The applicable box below must be completed
when this page is folded over.*

TRANSFER TO NEW PAGE

New page number transferred to: _____

Remaining quantity being transferred: _____

Date of transfer: _____

Nurse/LP making transfer: _____

TRANSFER TO DIFFERENT LOCATION

New location transferred to: _____

New page number transferred to: _____

Remaining quantity being transferred: _____

Date of transfer: _____

Nurse/LP making transfer: _____

Nurse/LP receiving transfer: _____

SURRENDER TO PERSON

Remaining quantity being surrendered: _____

Nurse/LP making surrender: _____

Person Surrendered To
Printed Name: _____
Signature: _____
- Patient - Responsible Party - Nurse/LP - Administrator - (circle one)

DEPLETION OF DRUG / MED
NONE REMAINING – PAGE FINISHED

Date completed: _____

Nurse/LP completing: _____

CONTROLLED DRUG / MED SUPPLY

Drug / Med Name:

Drug / Med Given			Present Balance	In From Pharmacy	Patient's Name	Prescriber's Name	Nurse/LP's Signature
Date	Time	Dose					

Two Nurse/LPs must witness and sign the destruction / waste of any controlled drugs / meds.
When folding pages over, the disposition of drugs / meds must be documented appropriately.

CONTROLLED DRUG / MED DISPOSITION

The applicable box below must be completed
when this page is folded over.

TRANSFER TO NEW PAGE

New page number transferred to: _____

Remaining quantity being transferred: _____

Date of transfer: _____

Nurse/LP making transfer: _____

TRANSFER TO DIFFERENT LOCATION

New location transferred to: _____

New page number transferred to: _____

Remaining quantity being transferred: _____

Date of transfer: _____

Nurse/LP making transfer: _____

Nurse/LP receiving transfer: _____

SURRENDER TO PERSON

Remaining quantity being surrendered: _____

Nurse/LP making surrender: _____

Person Surrendered To
Printed Name: _____
Signature: _____
- Patient - Responsible Party - Nurse/LP - Administrator - (circle one)

DEPLETION OF DRUG / MED
NONE REMAINING – PAGE FINISHED

Date completed: _____

Nurse/LP completing: _____

CONTROLLED DRUG / MED SUPPLY

Drug / Med Name: _____ Page No: **79**

Drug / Med Given			Present Balance	In From Pharmacy	Patient's Name	Prescriber's Name	Nurse/LP's Signature
Date	Time	Dose					

Two Nurse/LPs must witness and sign the destruction / waste of any controlled drugs / meds.
When folding pages over, the disposition of drugs / meds must be documented appropriately.

CONTROLLED DRUG / MED DISPOSITION

*The applicable box below must be completed
when this page is folded over.*

TRANSFER TO NEW PAGE

New page number transferred to: _____

Remaining quantity being transferred: _____

Date of transfer: _____

Nurse/LP making transfer: _____

TRANSFER TO DIFFERENT LOCATION

New location transferred to: _____

New page number transferred to: _____

Remaining quantity being transferred: _____

Date of transfer: _____

Nurse/LP making transfer: _____

Nurse/LP receiving transfer: _____

SURRENDER TO PERSON

Remaining quantity being surrendered: _____

Nurse/LP making surrender: _____

Person Surrendered To
Printed Name: _____
Signature: _____
- Patient - Responsible Party - Nurse/LP - Administrator - (circle one)

DEPLETION OF DRUG / MED
NONE REMAINING – PAGE FINISHED

Date completed: _____

Nurse/LP completing: _____

CONTROLLED DRUG / MED SUPPLY

Drug / Med Name: _____ Page No: **80**

Drug / Med Given			Present Balance	In From Pharmacy	Patient's Name	Prescriber's Name	Nurse/LP's Signature
Date	Time	Dose					

Two Nurse/LPs must witness and sign the destruction / waste of any controlled drugs / meds.
When folding pages over, the disposition of drugs / meds must be documented appropriately.

CONTROLLED DRUG / MED DISPOSITION

The applicable box below must be completed
when this page is folded over.

TRANSFER TO NEW PAGE

New page number transferred to: _____

Remaining quantity being transferred: _____

Date of transfer: _____

Nurse/LP making transfer: _____

TRANSFER TO DIFFERENT LOCATION

New location transferred to: _____

New page number transferred to: _____

Remaining quantity being transferred: _____

Date of transfer: _____

Nurse/LP making transfer: _____

Nurse/LP receiving transfer: _____

SURRENDER TO PERSON

Remaining quantity being surrendered: _____

Nurse/LP making surrender: _____

Person Surrendered To
Printed Name: _____
Signature: _____
- Patient - Responsible Party - Nurse/LP - Administrator - (circle one)

DEPLETION OF DRUG / MED
NONE REMAINING – PAGE FINISHED

Date completed: _____

Nurse/LP completing: _____

CONTROLLED DRUG / MED SUPPLY

Drug / Med Name: ⬚⬚⬚⬚⬚⬚⬚⬚⬚⬚⬚⬚⬚⬚⬚⬚⬚⬚⬚⬚⬚⬚⬚⬚⬚⬚⬚⬚⬚⬚⬚⬚ Page No: **81**

Drug / Med Given			Present Balance	In From Pharmacy	Patient's Name	Prescriber's Name	Nurse/LP's Signature
Date	Time	Dose					

Two Nurse/LPs must witness and sign the destruction / waste of any controlled drugs / meds.
When folding pages over, the disposition of drugs / meds must be documented appropriately.

CONTROLLED DRUG / MED DISPOSITION

The applicable box below must be completed
when this page is folded over.

TRANSFER TO NEW PAGE

New page number transferred to: _____

Remaining quantity being transferred: _____

Date of transfer: _____

Nurse/LP making transfer: _____

TRANSFER TO DIFFERENT LOCATION

New location transferred to: _____

New page number transferred to: _____

Remaining quantity being transferred: _____

Date of transfer: _____

Nurse/LP making transfer: _____

Nurse/LP receiving transfer: _____

SURRENDER TO PERSON

Remaining quantity being surrendered: _____

Nurse/LP making surrender: _____

Person Surrendered To
Printed Name: _____
Signature: _____
- Patient - Responsible Party - Nurse/LP - Administrator - (circle one)

DEPLETION OF DRUG / MED
NONE REMAINING – PAGE FINISHED

Date completed: _____

Nurse/LP completing: _____

CONTROLLED DRUG / MED SUPPLY

Drug / Med Name:

Drug / Med Given			Present Balance	In From Pharmacy	Patient's Name	Prescriber's Name	Nurse/LP's Signature
Date	Time	Dose					

Two Nurse/LPs must witness and sign the destruction / waste of any controlled drugs / meds.
When folding pages over, the disposition of drugs / meds must be documented appropriately.

CONTROLLED DRUG / MED DISPOSITION

*The applicable box below must be completed
when this page is folded over.*

TRANSFER TO NEW PAGE

New page number transferred to: _____

Remaining quantity being transferred: _____

Date of transfer: _____

Nurse/LP making transfer: _____

TRANSFER TO DIFFERENT LOCATION

New location transferred to: _____

New page number transferred to: _____

Remaining quantity being transferred: _____

Date of transfer: _____

Nurse/LP making transfer: _____

Nurse/LP receiving transfer: _____

SURRENDER TO PERSON

Remaining quantity being surrendered: _____

Nurse/LP making surrender: _____

Person Surrendered To
Printed Name: _____
Signature: _____
- Patient - Responsible Party - Nurse/LP - Administrator - (circle one)

DEPLETION OF DRUG / MED
NONE REMAINING – PAGE FINISHED

Date completed: _____

Nurse/LP completing: _____

CONTROLLED DRUG / MED SUPPLY

Drug / Med Name: Page No: **83**

Drug / Med Given			Present Balance	In From Pharmacy	Patient's Name	Prescriber's Name	Nurse/LP's Signature
Date	Time	Dose					

Two Nurse/LPs must witness and sign the destruction / waste of any controlled drugs / meds.
When folding pages over, the disposition of drugs / meds must be documented appropriately.

CONTROLLED DRUG / MED DISPOSITION

*The applicable box below must be completed
when this page is folded over.*

TRANSFER TO NEW PAGE

New page number transferred to: _____

Remaining quantity being transferred: _____

Date of transfer: _____

Nurse/LP making transfer: _____

TRANSFER TO DIFFERENT LOCATION

New location transferred to: _____

New page number transferred to: _____

Remaining quantity being transferred: _____

Date of transfer: _____

Nurse/LP making transfer: _____

Nurse/LP receiving transfer: _____

SURRENDER TO PERSON

Remaining quantity being surrendered: _____

Nurse/LP making surrender: _____

Person Surrendered To
Printed Name: _____
Signature: _____
- Patient - Responsible Party - Nurse/LP - Administrator - (circle one)

DEPLETION OF DRUG / MED
NONE REMAINING – PAGE FINISHED

Date completed: _____

Nurse/LP completing: _____

CONTROLLED DRUG / MED SUPPLY

Drug / Med Name:

Drug / Med Given			Present Balance	In From Pharmacy	Patient's Name	Prescriber's Name	Nurse/LP's Signature
Date	Time	Dose					

Two Nurse/LPs must witness and sign the destruction / waste of any controlled drugs / meds.
When folding pages over, the disposition of drugs / meds must be documented appropriately.

CONTROLLED DRUG / MED DISPOSITION

*The applicable box below must be completed
when this page is folded over.*

TRANSFER TO NEW PAGE

New page number transferred to: _____

Remaining quantity being transferred: _____

Date of transfer: _____

Nurse/LP making transfer: _____

TRANSFER TO DIFFERENT LOCATION

New location transferred to: _____

New page number transferred to: _____

Remaining quantity being transferred: _____

Date of transfer: _____

Nurse/LP making transfer: _____

Nurse/LP receiving transfer: _____

SURRENDER TO PERSON

Remaining quantity being surrendered: _____

Nurse/LP making surrender: _____

Person Surrendered To
Printed Name: _____
Signature: _____
- Patient - Responsible Party - Nurse/LP - Administrator - (circle one)

DEPLETION OF DRUG / MED
NONE REMAINING – PAGE FINISHED

Date completed: _____

Nurse/LP completing: _____

CONTROLLED DRUG / MED SUPPLY

Drug / Med Name: Page No: **85**

Drug / Med Given			Present Balance	In From Pharmacy	Patient's Name	Prescriber's Name	Nurse/LP's Signature
Date	Time	Dose					

Two Nurse/LPs must witness and sign the destruction / waste of any controlled drugs / meds.
When folding pages over, the disposition of drugs / meds must be documented appropriately.

CONTROLLED DRUG / MED DISPOSITION

*The applicable box below must be completed
when this page is folded over.*

TRANSFER TO NEW PAGE

New page number transferred to: _____

Remaining quantity being transferred: _____

Date of transfer: _____

Nurse/LP making transfer: _____

TRANSFER TO DIFFERENT LOCATION

New location transferred to: _____

New page number transferred to: _____

Remaining quantity being transferred: _____

Date of transfer: _____

Nurse/LP making transfer: _____

Nurse/LP receiving transfer: _____

SURRENDER TO PERSON

Remaining quantity being surrendered: _____

Nurse/LP making surrender: _____

Person Surrendered To
Printed Name: _____
Signature: _____
- Patient - Responsible Party - Nurse/LP - Administrator - (circle one)

DEPLETION OF DRUG / MED
NONE REMAINING – PAGE FINISHED

Date completed: _____

Nurse/LP completing: _____

CONTROLLED DRUG / MED SUPPLY

Drug / Med Name:

Drug / Med Given			Present Balance	In From Pharmacy	Patient's Name	Prescriber's Name	Nurse/LP's Signature
Date	Time	Dose					

Two Nurse/LPs must witness and sign the destruction / waste of any controlled drugs / meds.
When folding pages over, the disposition of drugs / meds must be documented appropriately.

CONTROLLED DRUG / MED DISPOSITION

The applicable box below must be completed when this page is folded over.

TRANSFER TO NEW PAGE

New page number transferred to: _____

Remaining quantity being transferred: _____

Date of transfer: _____

Nurse/LP making transfer: _____

TRANSFER TO DIFFERENT LOCATION

New location transferred to: _____

New page number transferred to: _____

Remaining quantity being transferred: _____

Date of transfer: _____

Nurse/LP making transfer: _____

Nurse/LP receiving transfer: _____

SURRENDER TO PERSON

Remaining quantity being surrendered: _____

Nurse/LP making surrender: _____

Person Surrendered To
Printed Name: _____
Signature: _____
- Patient - Responsible Party - Nurse/LP - Administrator - (circle one)

DEPLETION OF DRUG / MED
NONE REMAINING – PAGE FINISHED

Date completed: _____

Nurse/LP completing: _____

CONTROLLED DRUG / MED SUPPLY

Drug / Med Name:

Drug / Med Given			Present Balance	In From Pharmacy	Patient's Name	Prescriber's Name	Nurse/LP's Signature
Date	Time	Dose					

Two Nurse/LPs must witness and sign the destruction / waste of any controlled drugs / meds.
When folding pages over, the disposition of drugs / meds must be documented appropriately.

CONTROLLED DRUG / MED DISPOSITION

*The applicable box below must be completed
when this page is folded over.*

TRANSFER TO NEW PAGE

New page number transferred to: _____

Remaining quantity being transferred: _____

Date of transfer: _____

Nurse/LP making transfer: _____

TRANSFER TO DIFFERENT LOCATION

New location transferred to: _____

New page number transferred to: _____

Remaining quantity being transferred: _____

Date of transfer: _____

Nurse/LP making transfer: _____

Nurse/LP receiving transfer: _____

SURRENDER TO PERSON

Remaining quantity being surrendered: _____

Nurse/LP making surrender: _____

Person Surrendered To
Printed Name: _____
Signature: _____
- Patient - Responsible Party - Nurse/LP - Administrator - (circle one)

DEPLETION OF DRUG / MED
NONE REMAINING – PAGE FINISHED

Date completed: _____

Nurse/LP completing: _____

CONTROLLED DRUG / MED SUPPLY

Drug / Med Name: Page No: **88**

Drug / Med Given			Present Balance	In From Pharmacy	Patient's Name	Prescriber's Name	Nurse/LP's Signature
Date	Time	Dose					

Two Nurse/LPs must witness and sign the destruction / waste of any controlled drugs / meds.
When folding pages over, the disposition of drugs / meds must be documented appropriately.

CONTROLLED DRUG / MED DISPOSITION

*The applicable box below must be completed
when this page is folded over.*

TRANSFER TO NEW PAGE

New page number transferred to: _____

Remaining quantity being transferred: _____

Date of transfer: _____

Nurse/LP making transfer: _____

TRANSFER TO DIFFERENT LOCATION

New location transferred to: _____

New page number transferred to: _____

Remaining quantity being transferred: _____

Date of transfer: _____

Nurse/LP making transfer: _____

Nurse/LP receiving transfer: _____

SURRENDER TO PERSON

Remaining quantity being surrendered: _____

Nurse/LP making surrender: _____

Person Surrendered To
Printed Name: _____
Signature: _____
- Patient - Responsible Party - Nurse/LP - Administrator -   (circle one)

DEPLETION OF DRUG / MED
NONE REMAINING – PAGE FINISHED

Date completed: _____

Nurse/LP completing: _____

CONTROLLED DRUG / MED SUPPLY

Drug / Med Name: _____ Page No: **89**

Drug / Med Given			Present Balance	In From Pharmacy	Patient's Name	Prescriber's Name	Nurse/LP's Signature
Date	Time	Dose					

Two Nurse/LPs must witness and sign the destruction / waste of any controlled drugs / meds.
When folding pages over, the disposition of drugs / meds must be documented appropriately.

CONTROLLED DRUG / MED DISPOSITION

*The applicable box below must be completed
when this page is folded over.*

TRANSFER TO NEW PAGE

New page number transferred to: _____

Remaining quantity being transferred: _____

Date of transfer: _____

Nurse/LP making transfer: _____

TRANSFER TO DIFFERENT LOCATION

New location transferred to: _____

New page number transferred to: _____

Remaining quantity being transferred: _____

Date of transfer: _____

Nurse/LP making transfer: _____

Nurse/LP receiving transfer: _____

SURRENDER TO PERSON

Remaining quantity being surrendered: _____

Nurse/LP making surrender: _____

Person Surrendered To
Printed Name: _____
Signature: _____
- Patient - Responsible Party - Nurse/LP - Administrator - (circle one)

DEPLETION OF DRUG / MED
NONE REMAINING – PAGE FINISHED

Date completed: _____

Nurse/LP completing: _____

CONTROLLED DRUG / MED SUPPLY

Drug / Med Name:

Drug / Med Given			Present Balance	In From Pharmacy	Patient's Name	Prescriber's Name	Nurse/LP's Signature
Date	Time	Dose					

Two Nurse/LPs must witness and sign the destruction / waste of any controlled drugs / meds.
When folding pages over, the disposition of drugs / meds must be documented appropriately.

CONTROLLED DRUG / MED DISPOSITION

*The applicable box below must be completed
when this page is folded over.*

TRANSFER TO NEW PAGE

New page number transferred to: _____

Remaining quantity being transferred: _____

Date of transfer: _____

Nurse/LP making transfer: _____

TRANSFER TO DIFFERENT LOCATION

New location transferred to: _____

New page number transferred to: _____

Remaining quantity being transferred: _____

Date of transfer: _____

Nurse/LP making transfer: _____

Nurse/LP receiving transfer: _____

SURRENDER TO PERSON

Remaining quantity being surrendered: _____

Nurse/LP making surrender: _____

Person Surrendered To
Printed Name: _____
Signature: _____
- Patient - Responsible Party - Nurse/LP - Administrator - (circle one)

DEPLETION OF DRUG / MED
NONE REMAINING – PAGE FINISHED

Date completed: _____

Nurse/LP completing: _____

CONTROLLED DRUG / MED SUPPLY

Drug / Med Name: Page No: **91**

Drug / Med Given			Present Balance	In From Pharmacy	Patient's Name	Prescriber's Name	Nurse/LP's Signature
Date	Time	Dose					

Two Nurse/LPs must witness and sign the destruction / waste of any controlled drugs / meds.
When folding pages over, the disposition of drugs / meds must be documented appropriately.

CONTROLLED DRUG / MED DISPOSITION

*The applicable box below must be completed
when this page is folded over.*

TRANSFER TO NEW PAGE

New page number transferred to: _____

Remaining quantity being transferred: _____

Date of transfer: _____

Nurse/LP making transfer: _____

TRANSFER TO DIFFERENT LOCATION

New location transferred to: _____

New page number transferred to: _____

Remaining quantity being transferred: _____

Date of transfer: _____

Nurse/LP making transfer: _____

Nurse/LP receiving transfer: _____

SURRENDER TO PERSON

Remaining quantity being surrendered: _____

Nurse/LP making surrender: _____

Person Surrendered To
Printed Name: _____
Signature: _____
- Patient - Responsible Party - Nurse/LP - Administrator - (circle one)

DEPLETION OF DRUG / MED
NONE REMAINING – PAGE FINISHED

Date completed: _____

Nurse/LP completing: _____

CONTROLLED DRUG / MED SUPPLY

Drug / Med Name: _____ Page No: **92**

Drug / Med Given			Present Balance	In From Pharmacy	Patient's Name	Prescriber's Name	Nurse/LP's Signature
Date	Time	Dose					

Two Nurse/LPs must witness and sign the destruction / waste of any controlled drugs / meds.
When folding pages over, the disposition of drugs / meds must be documented appropriately.

CONTROLLED DRUG / MED DISPOSITION

*The applicable box below must be completed
when this page is folded over.*

TRANSFER TO NEW PAGE

New page number transferred to: _____

Remaining quantity being transferred: _____

Date of transfer: _____

Nurse/LP making transfer: _____

TRANSFER TO DIFFERENT LOCATION

New location transferred to: _____

New page number transferred to: _____

Remaining quantity being transferred: _____

Date of transfer: _____

Nurse/LP making transfer: _____

Nurse/LP receiving transfer: _____

SURRENDER TO PERSON

Remaining quantity being surrendered: _____

Nurse/LP making surrender: _____

Person Surrendered To
Printed Name: _____
Signature: _____
- Patient - Responsible Party - Nurse/LP - Administrator - (circle one)

DEPLETION OF DRUG / MED
NONE REMAINING – PAGE FINISHED

Date completed: _____

Nurse/LP completing: _____

CONTROLLED DRUG / MED SUPPLY

Drug / Med Name:

Drug / Med Given			Present Balance	In From Pharmacy	Patient's Name	Prescriber's Name	Nurse/LP's Signature
Date	Time	Dose					

Two Nurse/LPs must witness and sign the destruction / waste of any controlled drugs / meds.
When folding pages over, the disposition of drugs / meds must be documented appropriately.

CONTROLLED DRUG / MED DISPOSITION

*The applicable box below must be completed
when this page is folded over.*

TRANSFER TO NEW PAGE

New page number transferred to: _____

Remaining quantity being transferred: _____

Date of transfer: _____

Nurse/LP making transfer: _____

TRANSFER TO DIFFERENT LOCATION

New location transferred to: _____

New page number transferred to: _____

Remaining quantity being transferred: _____

Date of transfer: _____

Nurse/LP making transfer: _____

Nurse/LP receiving transfer: _____

SURRENDER TO PERSON

Remaining quantity being surrendered: _____

Nurse/LP making surrender: _____

Person Surrendered To

Printed Name: _____

Signature: _____

- Patient - Responsible Party - Nurse/LP - Administrator -
(circle one)

DEPLETION OF DRUG / MED
NONE REMAINING – PAGE FINISHED

Date completed: _____

Nurse/LP completing: _____

CONTROLLED DRUG / MED SUPPLY

Drug / Med Name: Page No:

Drug / Med Given			Present Balance	In From Pharmacy	Patient's Name	Prescriber's Name	Nurse/LP's Signature
Date	Time	Dose					

Two Nurse/LPs must witness and sign the destruction / waste of any controlled drugs / meds.
When folding pages over, the disposition of drugs / meds must be documented appropriately.

CONTROLLED DRUG / MED DISPOSITION

*The applicable box below must be completed
when this page is folded over.*

TRANSFER TO NEW PAGE

New page number transferred to: _____

Remaining quantity being transferred: _____

Date of transfer: _____

Nurse/LP making transfer: _____

TRANSFER TO DIFFERENT LOCATION

New location transferred to: _____

New page number transferred to: _____

Remaining quantity being transferred: _____

Date of transfer: _____

Nurse/LP making transfer: _____

Nurse/LP receiving transfer: _____

SURRENDER TO PERSON

Remaining quantity being surrendered: _____

Nurse/LP making surrender: _____

Person Surrendered To
Printed Name: _____
Signature: _____
- Patient - Responsible Party - Nurse/LP - Administrator -   (circle one)

DEPLETION OF DRUG / MED
NONE REMAINING – PAGE FINISHED

Date completed: _____

Nurse/LP completing: _____

CONTROLLED DRUG / MED SUPPLY

Drug / Med Name: Page No: **95**

Drug / Med Given			Present Balance	In From Pharmacy	Patient's Name	Prescriber's Name	Nurse/LP's Signature
Date	Time	Dose					

Two Nurse/LPs must witness and sign the destruction / waste of any controlled drugs / meds.
When folding pages over, the disposition of drugs / meds must be documented appropriately.

CONTROLLED DRUG / MED DISPOSITION

*The applicable box below must be completed
when this page is folded over.*

TRANSFER TO NEW PAGE

New page number transferred to: _____

Remaining quantity being transferred: _____

Date of transfer: _____

Nurse/LP making transfer: _____

TRANSFER TO DIFFERENT LOCATION

New location transferred to: _____

New page number transferred to: _____

Remaining quantity being transferred: _____

Date of transfer: _____

Nurse/LP making transfer: _____

Nurse/LP receiving transfer: _____

SURRENDER TO PERSON

Remaining quantity being surrendered: _____

Nurse/LP making surrender: _____

Person Surrendered To
Printed Name: _____
Signature: _____
- Patient - Responsible Party - Nurse/LP - Administrator - (circle one)

DEPLETION OF DRUG / MED
NONE REMAINING – PAGE FINISHED

Date completed: _____

Nurse/LP completing: _____

CONTROLLED DRUG / MED SUPPLY

| Drug / Med Name: | | | | | | | Page No: | 96 |

Drug / Med Given			Present Balance	In From Pharmacy	Patient's Name	Prescriber's Name	Nurse/LP's Signature
Date	Time	Dose					

Two Nurse/LPs must witness and sign the destruction / waste of any controlled drugs / meds.
When folding pages over, the disposition of drugs / meds must be documented appropriately.

CONTROLLED DRUG / MED DISPOSITION

The applicable box below must be completed
when this page is folded over.

TRANSFER TO NEW PAGE

New page number transferred to: _____

Remaining quantity being transferred: _____

Date of transfer: _____

Nurse/LP making transfer: _____

TRANSFER TO DIFFERENT LOCATION

New location transferred to: _____

New page number transferred to: _____

Remaining quantity being transferred: _____

Date of transfer: _____

Nurse/LP making transfer: _____

Nurse/LP receiving transfer: _____

SURRENDER TO PERSON

Remaining quantity being surrendered: _____

Nurse/LP making surrender: _____

Person Surrendered To
Printed Name: _____
Signature: _____
- Patient - Responsible Party - Nurse/LP - Administrator - (circle one)

DEPLETION OF DRUG / MED
NONE REMAINING – PAGE FINISHED

Date completed: _____

Nurse/LP completing: _____

CONTROLLED DRUG / MED SUPPLY

Drug / Med Name: Page No: **97**

Drug / Med Given			Present Balance	In From Pharmacy	Patient's Name	Prescriber's Name	Nurse/LP's Signature
Date	Time	Dose					

Two Nurse/LPs must witness and sign the destruction / waste of any controlled drugs / meds.
When folding pages over, the disposition of drugs / meds must be documented appropriately.

CONTROLLED DRUG / MED DISPOSITION

The applicable box below must be completed
when this page is folded over.

TRANSFER TO NEW PAGE

New page number transferred to: _____

Remaining quantity being transferred: _____

Date of transfer: _____

Nurse/LP making transfer: _____

TRANSFER TO DIFFERENT LOCATION

New location transferred to: _____

New page number transferred to: _____

Remaining quantity being transferred: _____

Date of transfer: _____

Nurse/LP making transfer: _____

Nurse/LP receiving transfer: _____

SURRENDER TO PERSON

Remaining quantity being surrendered: _____

Nurse/LP making surrender: _____

Person Surrendered To
Printed Name: _____
Signature: _____
- Patient - Responsible Party - Nurse/LP - Administrator - (circle one)

DEPLETION OF DRUG / MED
NONE REMAINING – PAGE FINISHED

Date completed: _____

Nurse/LP completing: _____

CONTROLLED DRUG / MED SUPPLY

Drug / Med Name: _____   Page No: **98**

Drug / Med Given			Present Balance	In From Pharmacy	Patient's Name	Prescriber's Name	Nurse/LP's Signature
Date	Time	Dose					

Two Nurse/LPs must witness and sign the destruction / waste of any controlled drugs / meds.
When folding pages over, the disposition of drugs / meds must be documented appropriately.

CONTROLLED DRUG / MED DISPOSITION

*The applicable box below must be completed
when this page is folded over.*

TRANSFER TO NEW PAGE

New page number transferred to: _____

Remaining quantity being transferred: _____

Date of transfer: _____

Nurse/LP making transfer: _____

TRANSFER TO DIFFERENT LOCATION

New location transferred to: _____

New page number transferred to: _____

Remaining quantity being transferred: _____

Date of transfer: _____

Nurse/LP making transfer: _____

Nurse/LP receiving transfer: _____

SURRENDER TO PERSON

Remaining quantity being surrendered: _____

Nurse/LP making surrender: _____

Person Surrendered To
Printed Name: _____
Signature: _____
- Patient - Responsible Party - Nurse/LP - Administrator - (circle one)

DEPLETION OF DRUG / MED
NONE REMAINING – PAGE FINISHED

Date completed: _____

Nurse/LP completing: _____

CONTROLLED DRUG / MED SUPPLY

Drug / Med Name: Page No: **99**

Drug / Med Given			Present Balance	In From Pharmacy	Patient's Name	Prescriber's Name	Nurse/LP's Signature
Date	Time	Dose					

Two Nurse/LPs must witness and sign the destruction / waste of any controlled drugs / meds.
When folding pages over, the disposition of drugs / meds must be documented appropriately.

CONTROLLED DRUG / MED DISPOSITION

The applicable box below must be completed
when this page is folded over.

TRANSFER TO NEW PAGE

New page number transferred to: _____

Remaining quantity being transferred: _____

Date of transfer: _____

Nurse/LP making transfer: _____

TRANSFER TO DIFFERENT LOCATION

New location transferred to: _____

New page number transferred to: _____

Remaining quantity being transferred: _____

Date of transfer: _____

Nurse/LP making transfer: _____

Nurse/LP receiving transfer: _____

SURRENDER TO PERSON

Remaining quantity being surrendered: _____

Nurse/LP making surrender: _____

Person Surrendered To
Printed Name: _____
Signature: _____
- Patient - Responsible Party - Nurse/LP - Administrator - (circle one)

DEPLETION OF DRUG / MED
NONE REMAINING – PAGE FINISHED

Date completed: _____

Nurse/LP completing: _____

CONTROLLED DRUG / MED SUPPLY

Drug / Med Name: _____ Page No: **100**

Drug / Med Given			Present Balance	In From Pharmacy	Patient's Name	Prescriber's Name	Nurse/LP's Signature
Date	Time	Dose					

Two Nurse/LPs must witness and sign the destruction / waste of any controlled drugs / meds.
When folding pages over, the disposition of drugs / meds must be documented appropriately.

CONTROLLED DRUG / MED DISPOSITION

The applicable box below must be completed
when this page is folded over.

TRANSFER TO NEW PAGE

New page number transferred to: _____

Remaining quantity being transferred: _____

Date of transfer: _____

Nurse/LP making transfer: _____

TRANSFER TO DIFFERENT LOCATION

New location transferred to: _____

New page number transferred to: _____

Remaining quantity being transferred: _____

Date of transfer: _____

Nurse/LP making transfer: _____

Nurse/LP receiving transfer: _____

SURRENDER TO PERSON

Remaining quantity being surrendered: _____

Nurse/LP making surrender: _____

Person Surrendered To
Printed Name: _____
Signature: _____
- Patient - Responsible Party - Nurse/LP - Administrator -   (circle one)

DEPLETION OF DRUG / MED
NONE REMAINING – PAGE FINISHED

Date completed: _____

Nurse/LP completing: _____

CONTROLLED DRUG / MED SUPPLY

Drug / Med Name:

Drug / Med Given			Present Balance	In From Pharmacy	Patient's Name	Prescriber's Name	Nurse/LP's Signature
Date	Time	Dose					

Two Nurse/LPs must witness and sign the destruction / waste of any controlled drugs / meds.
When folding pages over, the disposition of drugs / meds must be documented appropriately.

CONTROLLED DRUG / MED DISPOSITION

*The applicable box below must be completed
when this page is folded over.*

TRANSFER TO NEW PAGE

New page number transferred to: _____

Remaining quantity being transferred: _____

Date of transfer: _____

Nurse/LP making transfer: _____

TRANSFER TO DIFFERENT LOCATION

New location transferred to: _____

New page number transferred to: _____

Remaining quantity being transferred: _____

Date of transfer: _____

Nurse/LP making transfer: _____

Nurse/LP receiving transfer: _____

SURRENDER TO PERSON

Remaining quantity being surrendered: _____

Nurse/LP making surrender: _____

Person Surrendered To
Printed Name: _____
Signature: _____
- Patient - Responsible Party - Nurse/LP - Administrator - (circle one)

DEPLETION OF DRUG / MED
NONE REMAINING – PAGE FINISHED

Date completed: _____

Nurse/LP completing: _____

CONTROLLED DRUG / MED SUPPLY

Drug / Med Name: Page No: **102**

Drug / Med Given			Present Balance	In From Pharmacy	Patient's Name	Prescriber's Name	Nurse/LP's Signature
Date	Time	Dose					

Two Nurse/LPs must witness and sign the destruction / waste of any controlled drugs / meds.
When folding pages over, the disposition of drugs / meds must be documented appropriately.

CONTROLLED DRUG / MED DISPOSITION

The applicable box below must be completed when this page is folded over.

TRANSFER TO NEW PAGE

New page number transferred to: _____

Remaining quantity being transferred: _____

Date of transfer: _____

Nurse/LP making transfer: _____

TRANSFER TO DIFFERENT LOCATION

New location transferred to: _____

New page number transferred to: _____

Remaining quantity being transferred: _____

Date of transfer: _____

Nurse/LP making transfer: _____

Nurse/LP receiving transfer: _____

SURRENDER TO PERSON

Remaining quantity being surrendered: _____

Nurse/LP making surrender: _____

Person Surrendered To
Printed Name: _____
Signature: _____
- Patient - Responsible Party - Nurse/LP - Administrator -   (circle one)

DEPLETION OF DRUG / MED
NONE REMAINING – PAGE FINISHED

Date completed: _____

Nurse/LP completing: _____

CONTROLLED DRUG / MED SUPPLY

Drug / Med Name: _____ Page No: **103**

Drug / Med Given			Present Balance	In From Pharmacy	Patient's Name	Prescriber's Name	Nurse/LP's Signature
Date	Time	Dose					

Two Nurse/LPs must witness and sign the destruction / waste of any controlled drugs / meds.
When folding pages over, the disposition of drugs / meds must be documented appropriately.

CONTROLLED DRUG / MED DISPOSITION

*The applicable box below must be completed
when this page is folded over.*

TRANSFER TO NEW PAGE

New page number transferred to: _____

Remaining quantity being transferred: _____

Date of transfer: _____

Nurse/LP making transfer: _____

TRANSFER TO DIFFERENT LOCATION

New location transferred to: _____

New page number transferred to: _____

Remaining quantity being transferred: _____

Date of transfer: _____

Nurse/LP making transfer: _____

Nurse/LP receiving transfer: _____

SURRENDER TO PERSON

Remaining quantity being surrendered: _____

Nurse/LP making surrender: _____

Person Surrendered To
Printed Name: _____
Signature: _____
- Patient - Responsible Party - Nurse/LP - Administrator - (circle one)

DEPLETION OF DRUG / MED
NONE REMAINING – PAGE FINISHED

Date completed: _____

Nurse/LP completing: _____

CONTROLLED DRUG / MED SUPPLY

Drug / Med Name:

Drug / Med Given			Present Balance	In From Pharmacy	Patient's Name	Prescriber's Name	Nurse/LP's Signature
Date	Time	Dose					

Two Nurse/LPs must witness and sign the destruction / waste of any controlled drugs / meds.
When folding pages over, the disposition of drugs / meds must be documented appropriately.

CONTROLLED DRUG / MED DISPOSITION

The applicable box below must be completed
when this page is folded over.

TRANSFER TO NEW PAGE

New page number transferred to: _____

Remaining quantity being transferred: _____

Date of transfer: _____

Nurse/LP making transfer: _____

TRANSFER TO DIFFERENT LOCATION

New location transferred to: _____

New page number transferred to: _____

Remaining quantity being transferred: _____

Date of transfer: _____

Nurse/LP making transfer: _____

Nurse/LP receiving transfer: _____

SURRENDER TO PERSON

Remaining quantity being surrendered: _____

Nurse/LP making surrender: _____

Person Surrendered To
Printed Name: _____
Signature: _____
- Patient - Responsible Party - Nurse/LP - Administrator -   (circle one)

DEPLETION OF DRUG / MED
NONE REMAINING – PAGE FINISHED

Date completed: _____

Nurse/LP completing: _____

CONTROLLED DRUG / MED SUPPLY

Drug / Med Name: _____ Page No: **105**

Drug / Med Given			Present Balance	In From Pharmacy	Patient's Name	Prescriber's Name	Nurse/LP's Signature
Date	Time	Dose					

Two Nurse/LPs must witness and sign the destruction / waste of any controlled drugs / meds.
When folding pages over, the disposition of drugs / meds must be documented appropriately.

CONTROLLED DRUG / MED DISPOSITION

The applicable box below must be completed when this page is folded over.

TRANSFER TO NEW PAGE

New page number transferred to: _____

Remaining quantity being transferred: _____

Date of transfer: _____

Nurse/LP making transfer: _____

TRANSFER TO DIFFERENT LOCATION

New location transferred to: _____

New page number transferred to: _____

Remaining quantity being transferred: _____

Date of transfer: _____

Nurse/LP making transfer: _____

Nurse/LP receiving transfer: _____

SURRENDER TO PERSON

Remaining quantity being surrendered: _____

Nurse/LP making surrender: _____

Person Surrendered To
Printed Name: _____
Signature: _____
- Patient - Responsible Party - Nurse/LP - Administrator - (circle one)

DEPLETION OF DRUG / MED
NONE REMAINING – PAGE FINISHED

Date completed: _____

Nurse/LP completing: _____

CONTROLLED DRUG / MED SUPPLY

Drug / Med Name: Page No: **106**

Drug / Med Given			Present Balance	In From Pharmacy	Patient's Name	Prescriber's Name	Nurse/LP's Signature
Date	Time	Dose					

Two Nurse/LPs must witness and sign the destruction / waste of any controlled drugs / meds.
When folding pages over, the disposition of drugs / meds must be documented appropriately.

CONTROLLED DRUG / MED DISPOSITION

*The applicable box below must be completed
when this page is folded over.*

TRANSFER TO NEW PAGE

New page number transferred to: _____

Remaining quantity being transferred: _____

Date of transfer: _____

Nurse/LP making transfer: _____

TRANSFER TO DIFFERENT LOCATION

New location transferred to: _____

New page number transferred to: _____

Remaining quantity being transferred: _____

Date of transfer: _____

Nurse/LP making transfer: _____

Nurse/LP receiving transfer: _____

SURRENDER TO PERSON

Remaining quantity being surrendered: _____

Nurse/LP making surrender: _____

Person Surrendered To
Printed Name: _____
Signature: _____
- Patient - Responsible Party - Nurse/LP - Administrator -   (circle one)

DEPLETION OF DRUG / MED
NONE REMAINING – PAGE FINISHED

Date completed: _____

Nurse/LP completing: _____

CONTROLLED DRUG / MED SUPPLY

Drug / Med Name: Page No: **107**

Drug / Med Given			Present Balance	In From Pharmacy	Patient's Name	Prescriber's Name	Nurse/LP's Signature
Date	Time	Dose					

Two Nurse/LPs must witness and sign the destruction / waste of any controlled drugs / meds.
When folding pages over, the disposition of drugs / meds must be documented appropriately.

CONTROLLED DRUG / MED DISPOSITION

*The applicable box below must be completed
when this page is folded over.*

TRANSFER TO NEW PAGE

New page number transferred to: _____

Remaining quantity being transferred: _____

Date of transfer: _____

Nurse/LP making transfer: _____

TRANSFER TO DIFFERENT LOCATION

New location transferred to: _____

New page number transferred to: _____

Remaining quantity being transferred: _____

Date of transfer: _____

Nurse/LP making transfer: _____

Nurse/LP receiving transfer: _____

SURRENDER TO PERSON

Remaining quantity being surrendered: _____

Nurse/LP making surrender: _____

Person Surrendered To
Printed Name: _____
Signature: _____
- Patient - Responsible Party - Nurse/LP - Administrator - (circle one)

DEPLETION OF DRUG / MED
NONE REMAINING – PAGE FINISHED

Date completed: _____

Nurse/LP completing: _____

CONTROLLED DRUG / MED SUPPLY

Drug / Med Name:

Page No: **108**

Drug / Med Given			Present Balance	In From Pharmacy	Patient's Name	Prescriber's Name	Nurse/LP's Signature
Date	Time	Dose					

Two Nurse/LPs must witness and sign the destruction / waste of any controlled drugs / meds.
When folding pages over, the disposition of drugs / meds must be documented appropriately.

CONTROLLED DRUG / MED DISPOSITION

*The applicable box below must be completed
when this page is folded over.*

TRANSFER TO NEW PAGE

New page number transferred to: _____

Remaining quantity being transferred: _____

Date of transfer: _____

Nurse/LP making transfer: _____

TRANSFER TO DIFFERENT LOCATION

New location transferred to: _____

New page number transferred to: _____

Remaining quantity being transferred: _____

Date of transfer: _____

Nurse/LP making transfer: _____

Nurse/LP receiving transfer: _____

SURRENDER TO PERSON

Remaining quantity being surrendered: _____

Nurse/LP making surrender: _____

Person Surrendered To
Printed Name: _____
Signature: _____
- Patient - Responsible Party - Nurse/LP - Administrator - (circle one)

DEPLETION OF DRUG / MED
NONE REMAINING – PAGE FINISHED

Date completed: _____

Nurse/LP completing: _____

CONTROLLED DRUG / MED SUPPLY

Drug / Med Name: Page No: **109**

Drug / Med Given			Present Balance	In From Pharmacy	Patient's Name	Prescriber's Name	Nurse/LP's Signature
Date	Time	Dose					

Two Nurse/LPs must witness and sign the destruction / waste of any controlled drugs / meds.
When folding pages over, the disposition of drugs / meds must be documented appropriately.

CONTROLLED DRUG / MED DISPOSITION

The applicable box below must be completed
when this page is folded over.

TRANSFER TO NEW PAGE

New page number transferred to: _____

Remaining quantity being transferred: _____

Date of transfer: _____

Nurse/LP making transfer: _____

TRANSFER TO DIFFERENT LOCATION

New location transferred to: _____

New page number transferred to: _____

Remaining quantity being transferred: _____

Date of transfer: _____

Nurse/LP making transfer: _____

Nurse/LP receiving transfer: _____

SURRENDER TO PERSON

Remaining quantity being surrendered: _____

Nurse/LP making surrender: _____

Person Surrendered To
Printed Name: _____
Signature: _____
- Patient - Responsible Party - Nurse/LP - Administrator - (circle one)

DEPLETION OF DRUG / MED
NONE REMAINING – PAGE FINISHED

Date completed: _____

Nurse/LP completing: _____

CONTROLLED DRUG / MED SUPPLY

Drug / Med Name:

Drug / Med Given			Present Balance	In From Pharmacy	Patient's Name	Prescriber's Name	Nurse/LP's Signature
Date	Time	Dose					

Two Nurse/LPs must witness and sign the destruction / waste of any controlled drugs / meds.
When folding pages over, the disposition of drugs / meds must be documented appropriately.

CONTROLLED DRUG / MED DISPOSITION

The applicable box below must be completed when this page is folded over.

TRANSFER TO NEW PAGE

New page number transferred to: _____

Remaining quantity being transferred: _____

Date of transfer: _____

Nurse/LP making transfer: _____

TRANSFER TO DIFFERENT LOCATION

New location transferred to: _____

New page number transferred to: _____

Remaining quantity being transferred: _____

Date of transfer: _____

Nurse/LP making transfer: _____

Nurse/LP receiving transfer: _____

SURRENDER TO PERSON

Remaining quantity being surrendered: _____

Nurse/LP making surrender: _____

Person Surrendered To
Printed Name: _____
Signature: _____
- Patient - Responsible Party - Nurse/LP - Administrator - (circle one)

DEPLETION OF DRUG / MED
NONE REMAINING – PAGE FINISHED

Date completed: _____

Nurse/LP completing: _____

CONTROLLED DRUG / MED SUPPLY

Drug / Med Name: Page No: **111**

Drug / Med Given			Present Balance	In From Pharmacy	Patient's Name	Prescriber's Name	Nurse/LP's Signature
Date	Time	Dose					

Two Nurse/LPs must witness and sign the destruction / waste of any controlled drugs / meds.
When folding pages over, the disposition of drugs / meds must be documented appropriately.

CONTROLLED DRUG / MED DISPOSITION

The applicable box below must be completed
when this page is folded over.

TRANSFER TO NEW PAGE

New page number transferred to: _____

Remaining quantity being transferred: _____

Date of transfer: _____

Nurse/LP making transfer: _____

TRANSFER TO DIFFERENT LOCATION

New location transferred to: _____

New page number transferred to: _____

Remaining quantity being transferred: _____

Date of transfer: _____

Nurse/LP making transfer: _____

Nurse/LP receiving transfer: _____

SURRENDER TO PERSON

Remaining quantity being surrendered: _____

Nurse/LP making surrender: _____

Person Surrendered To
Printed Name: _____
Signature: _____
- Patient - Responsible Party - Nurse/LP - Administrator - (circle one)

DEPLETION OF DRUG / MED
NONE REMAINING – PAGE FINISHED

Date completed: _____

Nurse/LP completing: _____

CONTROLLED DRUG / MED SUPPLY

Drug / Med Name: Page No: **112**

Drug / Med Given			Present Balance	In From Pharmacy	Patient's Name	Prescriber's Name	Nurse/LP's Signature
Date	Time	Dose					

Two Nurse/LPs must witness and sign the destruction / waste of any controlled drugs / meds.
When folding pages over, the disposition of drugs / meds must be documented appropriately.

CONTROLLED DRUG / MED DISPOSITION

*The applicable box below must be completed
when this page is folded over.*

TRANSFER TO NEW PAGE

New page number transferred to: _____

Remaining quantity being transferred: _____

Date of transfer: _____

Nurse/LP making transfer: _____

TRANSFER TO DIFFERENT LOCATION

New location transferred to: _____

New page number transferred to: _____

Remaining quantity being transferred: _____

Date of transfer: _____

Nurse/LP making transfer: _____

Nurse/LP receiving transfer: _____

SURRENDER TO PERSON

Remaining quantity being surrendered: _____

Nurse/LP making surrender: _____

Person Surrendered To
Printed Name: _____
Signature: _____
- Patient - Responsible Party - Nurse/LP - Administrator - (circle one)

DEPLETION OF DRUG / MED
NONE REMAINING – PAGE FINISHED

Date completed: _____

Nurse/LP completing: _____

CONTROLLED DRUG / MED SUPPLY

Drug / Med Name: Page No: **113**

Date	Time	Dose	Present Balance	In From Pharmacy	Patient's Name	Prescriber's Name	Nurse/LP's Signature

Two Nurse/LPs must witness and sign the destruction / waste of any controlled drugs / meds.
When folding pages over, the disposition of drugs / meds must be documented appropriately.

CONTROLLED DRUG / MED DISPOSITION

*The applicable box below must be completed
when this page is folded over.*

TRANSFER TO NEW PAGE

New page number transferred to: _____

Remaining quantity being transferred: _____

Date of transfer: _____

Nurse/LP making transfer: _____

TRANSFER TO DIFFERENT LOCATION

New location transferred to: _____

New page number transferred to: _____

Remaining quantity being transferred: _____

Date of transfer: _____

Nurse/LP making transfer: _____

Nurse/LP receiving transfer: _____

SURRENDER TO PERSON

Remaining quantity being surrendered: _____

Nurse/LP making surrender: _____

Person Surrendered To
Printed Name: _____
Signature: _____
- Patient - Responsible Party - Nurse/LP - Administrator - (circle one)

DEPLETION OF DRUG / MED
NONE REMAINING – PAGE FINISHED

Date completed: _____

Nurse/LP completing: _____

CONTROLLED DRUG / MED SUPPLY

Drug / Med Name: Page No: **114**

Drug / Med Given			Present Balance	In From Pharmacy	Patient's Name	Prescriber's Name	Nurse/LP's Signature
Date	Time	Dose					

Two Nurse/LPs must witness and sign the destruction / waste of any controlled drugs / meds.
When folding pages over, the disposition of drugs / meds must be documented appropriately.

CONTROLLED DRUG / MED DISPOSITION

*The applicable box below must be completed
when this page is folded over.*

TRANSFER TO NEW PAGE

New page number transferred to: _____

Remaining quantity being transferred: _____

Date of transfer: _____

Nurse/LP making transfer: _____

TRANSFER TO DIFFERENT LOCATION

New location transferred to: _____

New page number transferred to: _____

Remaining quantity being transferred: _____

Date of transfer: _____

Nurse/LP making transfer: _____

Nurse/LP receiving transfer: _____

SURRENDER TO PERSON

Remaining quantity being surrendered: _____

Nurse/LP making surrender: _____

Person Surrendered To
Printed Name: _____
Signature: _____
- Patient - Responsible Party - Nurse/LP - Administrator - (circle one)

DEPLETION OF DRUG / MED
NONE REMAINING – PAGE FINISHED

Date completed: _____

Nurse/LP completing: _____

CONTROLLED DRUG / MED SUPPLY

Drug / Med Name:

Drug / Med Given			Present Balance	In From Pharmacy	Patient's Name	Prescriber's Name	Nurse/LP's Signature
Date	Time	Dose					

Two Nurse/LPs must witness and sign the destruction / waste of any controlled drugs / meds.
When folding pages over, the disposition of drugs / meds must be documented appropriately.

CONTROLLED DRUG / MED DISPOSITION

*The applicable box below must be completed
when this page is folded over.*

TRANSFER TO NEW PAGE

New page number transferred to: _____

Remaining quantity being transferred: _____

Date of transfer: _____

Nurse/LP making transfer: _____

TRANSFER TO DIFFERENT LOCATION

New location transferred to: _____

New page number transferred to: _____

Remaining quantity being transferred: _____

Date of transfer: _____

Nurse/LP making transfer: _____

Nurse/LP receiving transfer: _____

SURRENDER TO PERSON

Remaining quantity being surrendered: _____

Nurse/LP making surrender: _____

Person Surrendered To
Printed Name: _____
Signature: _____
- Patient - Responsible Party - Nurse/LP - Administrator - (circle one)

DEPLETION OF DRUG / MED
NONE REMAINING – PAGE FINISHED

Date completed: _____

Nurse/LP completing: _____

CONTROLLED DRUG / MED SUPPLY

Drug / Med Name: Page No: **116**

Drug / Med Given			Present Balance	In From Pharmacy	Patient's Name	Prescriber's Name	Nurse/LP's Signature
Date	Time	Dose					

Two Nurse/LPs must witness and sign the destruction / waste of any controlled drugs / meds.
When folding pages over, the disposition of drugs / meds must be documented appropriately.

CONTROLLED DRUG / MED DISPOSITION

The applicable box below must be completed
when this page is folded over.

TRANSFER TO NEW PAGE

New page number transferred to: _____

Remaining quantity being transferred: _____

Date of transfer: _____

Nurse/LP making transfer: _____

TRANSFER TO DIFFERENT LOCATION

New location transferred to: _____

New page number transferred to: _____

Remaining quantity being transferred: _____

Date of transfer: _____

Nurse/LP making transfer: _____

Nurse/LP receiving transfer: _____

SURRENDER TO PERSON

Remaining quantity being surrendered: _____

Nurse/LP making surrender: _____

Person Surrendered To
Printed Name: _____
Signature: _____
- Patient - Responsible Party - Nurse/LP - Administrator - (circle one)

DEPLETION OF DRUG / MED
NONE REMAINING – PAGE FINISHED

Date completed: _____

Nurse/LP completing: _____

CONTROLLED DRUG / MED SUPPLY

Drug / Med Name: Page No: **117**

Drug / Med Given			Present Balance	In From Pharmacy	Patient's Name	Prescriber's Name	Nurse/LP's Signature
Date	Time	Dose					

Two Nurse/LPs must witness and sign the destruction / waste of any controlled drugs / meds.
When folding pages over, the disposition of drugs / meds must be documented appropriately.

CONTROLLED DRUG / MED DISPOSITION

The applicable box below must be completed
when this page is folded over.

TRANSFER TO NEW PAGE

New page number transferred to: _____

Remaining quantity being transferred: _____

Date of transfer: _____

Nurse/LP making transfer: _____

TRANSFER TO DIFFERENT LOCATION

New location transferred to: _____

New page number transferred to: _____

Remaining quantity being transferred: _____

Date of transfer: _____

Nurse/LP making transfer: _____

Nurse/LP receiving transfer: _____

SURRENDER TO PERSON

Remaining quantity being surrendered: _____

Nurse/LP making surrender: _____

Person Surrendered To
Printed Name: _____
Signature: _____
- Patient - Responsible Party - Nurse/LP - Administrator - (circle one)

DEPLETION OF DRUG / MED
NONE REMAINING – PAGE FINISHED

Date completed: _____

Nurse/LP completing: _____

CONTROLLED DRUG / MED SUPPLY

Drug / Med Name: Page No: **118**

Drug / Med Given			Present Balance	In From Pharmacy	Patient's Name	Prescriber's Name	Nurse/LP's Signature
Date	Time	Dose					

Two Nurse/LPs must witness and sign the destruction / waste of any controlled drugs / meds.
When folding pages over, the disposition of drugs / meds must be documented appropriately.

CONTROLLED DRUG / MED DISPOSITION

The applicable box below must be completed
when this page is folded over.

TRANSFER TO NEW PAGE

New page number transferred to: _____

Remaining quantity being transferred: _____

Date of transfer: _____

Nurse/LP making transfer: _____

TRANSFER TO DIFFERENT LOCATION

New location transferred to: _____

New page number transferred to: _____

Remaining quantity being transferred: _____

Date of transfer: _____

Nurse/LP making transfer: _____

Nurse/LP receiving transfer: _____

SURRENDER TO PERSON

Remaining quantity being surrendered: _____

Nurse/LP making surrender: _____

Person Surrendered To
Printed Name: _____
Signature: _____
- Patient - Responsible Party - Nurse/LP - Administrator - (circle one)

DEPLETION OF DRUG / MED
NONE REMAINING – PAGE FINISHED

Date completed: _____

Nurse/LP completing: _____

CONTROLLED DRUG / MED SUPPLY

Drug / Med Name: Page No: **119**

Drug / Med Given			Present Balance	In From Pharmacy	Patient's Name	Prescriber's Name	Nurse/LP's Signature
Date	Time	Dose					

Two Nurse/LPs must witness and sign the destruction / waste of any controlled drugs / meds.
When folding pages over, the disposition of drugs / meds must be documented appropriately.

CONTROLLED DRUG / MED DISPOSITION

The applicable box below must be completed
when this page is folded over.

TRANSFER TO NEW PAGE

New page number transferred to: _____

Remaining quantity being transferred: _____

Date of transfer: _____

Nurse/LP making transfer: _____

TRANSFER TO DIFFERENT LOCATION

New location transferred to: _____

New page number transferred to: _____

Remaining quantity being transferred: _____

Date of transfer: _____

Nurse/LP making transfer: _____

Nurse/LP receiving transfer: _____

SURRENDER TO PERSON

Remaining quantity being surrendered: _____

Nurse/LP making surrender: _____

Person Surrendered To
Printed Name: _____
Signature: _____
- Patient - Responsible Party - Nurse/LP - Administrator - (circle one)

DEPLETION OF DRUG / MED
NONE REMAINING – PAGE FINISHED

Date completed: _____

Nurse/LP completing: _____

CONTROLLED DRUG / MED SUPPLY

Drug / Med Name: Page No: **120**

Drug / Med Given			Present Balance	In From Pharmacy	Patient's Name	Prescriber's Name	Nurse/LP's Signature
Date	Time	Dose					

Two Nurse/LPs must witness and sign the destruction / waste of any controlled drugs / meds.
When folding pages over, the disposition of drugs / meds must be documented appropriately.

CONTROLLED DRUG / MED DISPOSITION

*The applicable box below must be completed
when this page is folded over.*

TRANSFER TO NEW PAGE

New page number transferred to: _____

Remaining quantity being transferred: _____

Date of transfer: _____

Nurse/LP making transfer: _____

TRANSFER TO DIFFERENT LOCATION

New location transferred to: _____

New page number transferred to: _____

Remaining quantity being transferred: _____

Date of transfer: _____

Nurse/LP making transfer: _____

Nurse/LP receiving transfer: _____

SURRENDER TO PERSON

Remaining quantity being surrendered: _____

Nurse/LP making surrender: _____

Person Surrendered To
Printed Name: _____
Signature: _____
- Patient - Responsible Party - Nurse/LP - Administrator - (circle one)

DEPLETION OF DRUG / MED
NONE REMAINING – PAGE FINISHED

Date completed: _____

Nurse/LP completing: _____

CONTROLLED DRUG / MED SUPPLY

Drug / Med Name: _____

Drug / Med Given			Present Balance	In From Pharmacy	Patient's Name	Prescriber's Name	Nurse/LP's Signature
Date	Time	Dose					

Two Nurse/LPs must witness and sign the destruction / waste of any controlled drugs / meds.
When folding pages over, the disposition of drugs / meds must be documented appropriately.

CONTROLLED DRUG / MED DISPOSITION

The applicable box below must be completed
when this page is folded over.

TRANSFER TO NEW PAGE

New page number transferred to: _____

Remaining quantity being transferred: _____

Date of transfer: _____

Nurse/LP making transfer: _____

TRANSFER TO DIFFERENT LOCATION

New location transferred to: _____

New page number transferred to: _____

Remaining quantity being transferred: _____

Date of transfer: _____

Nurse/LP making transfer: _____

Nurse/LP receiving transfer: _____

SURRENDER TO PERSON

Remaining quantity being surrendered: _____

Nurse/LP making surrender: _____

Person Surrendered To
Printed Name: _____
Signature: _____
- Patient - Responsible Party - Nurse/LP - Administrator - (circle one)

DEPLETION OF DRUG / MED
NONE REMAINING – PAGE FINISHED

Date completed: _____

Nurse/LP completing: _____

CONTROLLED DRUG / MED SUPPLY

Drug / Med Name:						Page No:	**122**

Drug / Med Given			Present Balance	In From Pharmacy	Patient's Name	Prescriber's Name	Nurse/LP's Signature
Date	Time	Dose					

Two Nurse/LPs must witness and sign the destruction / waste of any controlled drugs / meds.
When folding pages over, the disposition of drugs / meds must be documented appropriately.

CONTROLLED DRUG / MED DISPOSITION

*The applicable box below must be completed
when this page is folded over.*

TRANSFER TO NEW PAGE

New page number transferred to: _____

Remaining quantity being transferred: _____

Date of transfer: _____

Nurse/LP making transfer: _____

TRANSFER TO DIFFERENT LOCATION

New location transferred to: _____

New page number transferred to: _____

Remaining quantity being transferred: _____

Date of transfer: _____

Nurse/LP making transfer: _____

Nurse/LP receiving transfer: _____

SURRENDER TO PERSON

Remaining quantity being surrendered: _____

Nurse/LP making surrender: _____

Person Surrendered To
Printed Name: _____
Signature: _____
- Patient - Responsible Party - Nurse/LP - Administrator - (circle one)

DEPLETION OF DRUG / MED
NONE REMAINING – PAGE FINISHED

Date completed: _____

Nurse/LP completing: _____

CONTROLLED DRUG / MED SUPPLY

Drug / Med Name:

Drug / Med Given			Present Balance	In From Pharmacy	Patient's Name	Prescriber's Name	Nurse/LP's Signature
Date	Time	Dose					

Two Nurse/LPs must witness and sign the destruction / waste of any controlled drugs / meds.
When folding pages over, the disposition of drugs / meds must be documented appropriately.

CONTROLLED DRUG / MED DISPOSITION

*The applicable box below must be completed
when this page is folded over.*

TRANSFER TO NEW PAGE

New page number transferred to: _____

Remaining quantity being transferred: _____

Date of transfer: _____

Nurse/LP making transfer: _____

TRANSFER TO DIFFERENT LOCATION

New location transferred to: _____

New page number transferred to: _____

Remaining quantity being transferred: _____

Date of transfer: _____

Nurse/LP making transfer: _____

Nurse/LP receiving transfer: _____

SURRENDER TO PERSON

Remaining quantity being surrendered: _____

Nurse/LP making surrender: _____

Person Surrendered To
Printed Name: _____
Signature: _____
- Patient - Responsible Party - Nurse/LP - Administrator - (circle one)

DEPLETION OF DRUG / MED
NONE REMAINING – PAGE FINISHED

Date completed: _____

Nurse/LP completing: _____

CONTROLLED DRUG / MED SUPPLY

Drug / Med Name: Page No: **124**

Drug / Med Given			Present Balance	In From Pharmacy	Patient's Name	Prescriber's Name	Nurse/LP's Signature
Date	Time	Dose					

Two Nurse/LPs must witness and sign the destruction / waste of any controlled drugs / meds.
When folding pages over, the disposition of drugs / meds must be documented appropriately.

CONTROLLED DRUG / MED DISPOSITION

*The applicable box below must be completed
when this page is folded over.*

TRANSFER TO NEW PAGE

New page number transferred to: _____

Remaining quantity being transferred: _____

Date of transfer: _____

Nurse/LP making transfer: _____

TRANSFER TO DIFFERENT LOCATION

New location transferred to: _____

New page number transferred to: _____

Remaining quantity being transferred: _____

Date of transfer: _____

Nurse/LP making transfer: _____

Nurse/LP receiving transfer: _____

SURRENDER TO PERSON

Remaining quantity being surrendered: _____

Nurse/LP making surrender: _____

Person Surrendered To
Printed Name: _____
Signature: _____
- Patient - Responsible Party - Nurse/LP - Administrator - (circle one)

DEPLETION OF DRUG / MED
NONE REMAINING – PAGE FINISHED

Date completed: _____

Nurse/LP completing: _____

CONTROLLED DRUG / MED SUPPLY

Drug / Med Name: Page No: **125**

Drug / Med Given			Present Balance	In From Pharmacy	Patient's Name	Prescriber's Name	Nurse/LP's Signature
Date	Time	Dose					

Two Nurse/LPs must witness and sign the destruction / waste of any controlled drugs / meds.
When folding pages over, the disposition of drugs / meds must be documented appropriately.

CONTROLLED DRUG / MED DISPOSITION

*The applicable box below must be completed
when this page is folded over.*

TRANSFER TO NEW PAGE

New page number transferred to: _____

Remaining quantity being transferred: _____

Date of transfer: _____

Nurse/LP making transfer: _____

TRANSFER TO DIFFERENT LOCATION

New location transferred to: _____

New page number transferred to: _____

Remaining quantity being transferred: _____

Date of transfer: _____

Nurse/LP making transfer: _____

Nurse/LP receiving transfer: _____

SURRENDER TO PERSON

Remaining quantity being surrendered: _____

Nurse/LP making surrender: _____

Person Surrendered To
Printed Name: _____
Signature: _____
- Patient - Responsible Party - Nurse/LP - Administrator - (circle one)

DEPLETION OF DRUG / MED
NONE REMAINING – PAGE FINISHED

Date completed: _____

Nurse/LP completing: _____

CONTROLLED DRUG / MED SUPPLY

Drug / Med Name:

Drug / Med Given			Present Balance	In From Pharmacy	Patient's Name	Prescriber's Name	Nurse/LP's Signature
Date	Time	Dose					

Two Nurse/LPs must witness and sign the destruction / waste of any controlled drugs / meds.
When folding pages over, the disposition of drugs / meds must be documented appropriately.

CONTROLLED DRUG / MED DISPOSITION

The applicable box below must be completed
when this page is folded over.

TRANSFER TO NEW PAGE

New page number transferred to: _____

Remaining quantity being transferred: _____

Date of transfer: _____

Nurse/LP making transfer: _____

TRANSFER TO DIFFERENT LOCATION

New location transferred to: _____

New page number transferred to: _____

Remaining quantity being transferred: _____

Date of transfer: _____

Nurse/LP making transfer: _____

Nurse/LP receiving transfer: _____

SURRENDER TO PERSON

Remaining quantity being surrendered: _____

Nurse/LP making surrender: _____

Person Surrendered To
Printed Name: _____
Signature: _____
- Patient - Responsible Party - Nurse/LP - Administrator - (circle one)

DEPLETION OF DRUG / MED
NONE REMAINING – PAGE FINISHED

Date completed: _____

Nurse/LP completing: _____

CONTROLLED DRUG / MED SUPPLY

Drug / Med Name: Page No: **127**

Drug / Med Given			Present Balance	In From Pharmacy	Patient's Name	Prescriber's Name	Nurse/LP's Signature
Date	Time	Dose					

Two Nurse/LPs must witness and sign the destruction / waste of any controlled drugs / meds.
When folding pages over, the disposition of drugs / meds must be documented appropriately.

CONTROLLED DRUG / MED DISPOSITION

*The applicable box below must be completed
when this page is folded over.*

TRANSFER TO NEW PAGE

New page number transferred to: _____

Remaining quantity being transferred: _____

Date of transfer: _____

Nurse/LP making transfer: _____

TRANSFER TO DIFFERENT LOCATION

New location transferred to: _____

New page number transferred to: _____

Remaining quantity being transferred: _____

Date of transfer: _____

Nurse/LP making transfer: _____

Nurse/LP receiving transfer: _____

SURRENDER TO PERSON

Remaining quantity being surrendered: _____

Nurse/LP making surrender: _____

Person Surrendered To
Printed Name: _____
Signature: _____
- Patient - Responsible Party - Nurse/LP - Administrator - (circle one)

DEPLETION OF DRUG / MED
NONE REMAINING – PAGE FINISHED

Date completed: _____

Nurse/LP completing: _____

CONTROLLED DRUG / MED SUPPLY

Drug / Med Name: _____ Page No: **128**

Drug / Med Given			Present Balance	In From Pharmacy	Patient's Name	Prescriber's Name	Nurse/LP's Signature
Date	Time	Dose					

Two Nurse/LPs must witness and sign the destruction / waste of any controlled drugs / meds.
When folding pages over, the disposition of drugs / meds must be documented appropriately.

CONTROLLED DRUG / MED DISPOSITION

The applicable box below must be completed
when this page is folded over.

TRANSFER TO NEW PAGE

New page number transferred to: _____

Remaining quantity being transferred: _____

Date of transfer: _____

Nurse/LP making transfer: _____

TRANSFER TO DIFFERENT LOCATION

New location transferred to: _____

New page number transferred to: _____

Remaining quantity being transferred: _____

Date of transfer: _____

Nurse/LP making transfer: _____

Nurse/LP receiving transfer: _____

SURRENDER TO PERSON

Remaining quantity being surrendered: _____

Nurse/LP making surrender: _____

Person Surrendered To
Printed Name: _____
Signature: _____
- Patient - Responsible Party - Nurse/LP - Administrator - (circle one)

DEPLETION OF DRUG / MED
NONE REMAINING – PAGE FINISHED

Date completed: _____

Nurse/LP completing: _____

CONTROLLED DRUG / MED SUPPLY

Drug / Med Name: Page No: **129**

Drug / Med Given			Present Balance	In From Pharmacy	Patient's Name	Prescriber's Name	Nurse/LP's Signature
Date	Time	Dose					

Two Nurse/LPs must witness and sign the destruction / waste of any controlled drugs / meds.
When folding pages over, the disposition of drugs / meds must be documented appropriately.

CONTROLLED DRUG / MED DISPOSITION

The applicable box below must be completed
when this page is folded over.

TRANSFER TO NEW PAGE

New page number transferred to: _____

Remaining quantity being transferred: _____

Date of transfer: _____

Nurse/LP making transfer: _____

TRANSFER TO DIFFERENT LOCATION

New location transferred to: _____

New page number transferred to: _____

Remaining quantity being transferred: _____

Date of transfer: _____

Nurse/LP making transfer: _____

Nurse/LP receiving transfer: _____

SURRENDER TO PERSON

Remaining quantity being surrendered: _____

Nurse/LP making surrender: _____

Person Surrendered To
Printed Name: _____
Signature: _____
- Patient - Responsible Party - Nurse/LP - Administrator -   (circle one)

DEPLETION OF DRUG / MED
NONE REMAINING – PAGE FINISHED

Date completed: _____

Nurse/LP completing: _____

CONTROLLED DRUG / MED SUPPLY

Drug / Med Name: Page No: **130**

Drug / Med Given			Present Balance	In From Pharmacy	Patient's Name	Prescriber's Name	Nurse/LP's Signature
Date	Time	Dose					

Two Nurse/LPs must witness and sign the destruction / waste of any controlled drugs / meds.
When folding pages over, the disposition of drugs / meds must be documented appropriately.

CONTROLLED DRUG / MED DISPOSITION

*The applicable box below must be completed
when this page is folded over.*

TRANSFER TO NEW PAGE

New page number transferred to: _____

Remaining quantity being transferred: _____

Date of transfer: _____

Nurse/LP making transfer: _____

TRANSFER TO DIFFERENT LOCATION

New location transferred to: _____

New page number transferred to: _____

Remaining quantity being transferred: _____

Date of transfer: _____

Nurse/LP making transfer: _____

Nurse/LP receiving transfer: _____

SURRENDER TO PERSON

Remaining quantity being surrendered: _____

Nurse/LP making surrender: _____

Person Surrendered To
Printed Name: _____
Signature: _____
- Patient - Responsible Party - Nurse/LP - Administrator - (circle one)

DEPLETION OF DRUG / MED
NONE REMAINING – PAGE FINISHED

Date completed: _____

Nurse/LP completing: _____

CONTROLLED DRUG / MED SUPPLY

Drug / Med Name:

Drug / Med Given			Present Balance	In From Pharmacy	Patient's Name	Prescriber's Name	Nurse/LP's Signature
Date	Time	Dose					

Two Nurse/LPs must witness and sign the destruction / waste of any controlled drugs / meds.
When folding pages over, the disposition of drugs / meds must be documented appropriately.

CONTROLLED DRUG / MED DISPOSITION

The applicable box below must be completed
when this page is folded over.

TRANSFER TO NEW PAGE

New page number transferred to: _____

Remaining quantity being transferred: _____

Date of transfer: _____

Nurse/LP making transfer: _____

TRANSFER TO DIFFERENT LOCATION

New location transferred to: _____

New page number transferred to: _____

Remaining quantity being transferred: _____

Date of transfer: _____

Nurse/LP making transfer: _____

Nurse/LP receiving transfer: _____

SURRENDER TO PERSON

Remaining quantity being surrendered: _____

Nurse/LP making surrender: _____

Person Surrendered To
Printed Name: _____
Signature: _____
- Patient - Responsible Party - Nurse/LP - Administrator - (circle one)

DEPLETION OF DRUG / MED
NONE REMAINING – PAGE FINISHED

Date completed: _____

Nurse/LP completing: _____

CONTROLLED DRUG / MED SUPPLY

Drug / Med Name:

Page No: **132**

Drug / Med Given			Present Balance	In From Pharmacy	Patient's Name	Prescriber's Name	Nurse/LP's Signature
Date	Time	Dose					

Two Nurse/LPs must witness and sign the destruction / waste of any controlled drugs / meds.
When folding pages over, the disposition of drugs / meds must be documented appropriately.

CONTROLLED DRUG / MED DISPOSITION

*The applicable box below must be completed
when this page is folded over.*

TRANSFER TO NEW PAGE

New page number transferred to: _____

Remaining quantity being transferred: _____

Date of transfer: _____

Nurse/LP making transfer: _____

TRANSFER TO DIFFERENT LOCATION

New location transferred to: _____

New page number transferred to: _____

Remaining quantity being transferred: _____

Date of transfer: _____

Nurse/LP making transfer: _____

Nurse/LP receiving transfer: _____

SURRENDER TO PERSON

Remaining quantity being surrendered: _____

Nurse/LP making surrender: _____

Person Surrendered To
Printed Name: _____
Signature: _____
- Patient - Responsible Party - Nurse/LP - Administrator - (circle one)

DEPLETION OF DRUG / MED
NONE REMAINING – PAGE FINISHED

Date completed: _____

Nurse/LP completing: _____

CONTROLLED DRUG / MED SUPPLY

Drug / Med Name: Page No: **133**

Drug / Med Given			Present Balance	In From Pharmacy	Patient's Name	Prescriber's Name	Nurse/LP's Signature
Date	Time	Dose					

Two Nurse/LPs must witness and sign the destruction / waste of any controlled drugs / meds.
When folding pages over, the disposition of drugs / meds must be documented appropriately.

CONTROLLED DRUG / MED DISPOSITION

The applicable box below must be completed
when this page is folded over.

TRANSFER TO NEW PAGE

New page number transferred to: _____

Remaining quantity being transferred: _____

Date of transfer: _____

Nurse/LP making transfer: _____

TRANSFER TO DIFFERENT LOCATION

New location transferred to: _____

New page number transferred to: _____

Remaining quantity being transferred: _____

Date of transfer: _____

Nurse/LP making transfer: _____

Nurse/LP receiving transfer: _____

SURRENDER TO PERSON

Remaining quantity being surrendered: _____

Nurse/LP making surrender: _____

Person Surrendered To
Printed Name: _____
Signature: _____
- Patient - Responsible Party - Nurse/LP - Administrator - (circle one)

DEPLETION OF DRUG / MED
NONE REMAINING – PAGE FINISHED

Date completed: _____

Nurse/LP completing: _____

CONTROLLED DRUG / MED SUPPLY

Drug / Med Name: Page No: **134**

Drug / Med Given			Present Balance	In From Pharmacy	Patient's Name	Prescriber's Name	Nurse/LP's Signature
Date	Time	Dose					

Two Nurse/LPs must witness and sign the destruction / waste of any controlled drugs / meds.
When folding pages over, the disposition of drugs / meds must be documented appropriately.

CONTROLLED DRUG / MED DISPOSITION

*The applicable box below must be completed
when this page is folded over.*

TRANSFER TO NEW PAGE

New page number transferred to: _____

Remaining quantity being transferred: _____

Date of transfer: _____

Nurse/LP making transfer: _____

TRANSFER TO DIFFERENT LOCATION

New location transferred to: _____

New page number transferred to: _____

Remaining quantity being transferred: _____

Date of transfer: _____

Nurse/LP making transfer: _____

Nurse/LP receiving transfer: _____

SURRENDER TO PERSON

Remaining quantity being surrendered: _____

Nurse/LP making surrender: _____

Person Surrendered To
Printed Name: _____
Signature: _____
- Patient - Responsible Party - Nurse/LP - Administrator - (circle one)

DEPLETION OF DRUG / MED
NONE REMAINING – PAGE FINISHED

Date completed: _____

Nurse/LP completing: _____

CONTROLLED DRUG / MED SUPPLY

Drug / Med Name: Page No: **135**

Drug / Med Given			Present Balance	In From Pharmacy	Patient's Name	Prescriber's Name	Nurse/LP's Signature
Date	Time	Dose					

Two Nurse/LPs must witness and sign the destruction / waste of any controlled drugs / meds.
When folding pages over, the disposition of drugs / meds must be documented appropriately.

CONTROLLED DRUG / MED DISPOSITION

*The applicable box below must be completed
when this page is folded over.*

TRANSFER TO NEW PAGE

New page number transferred to: _____

Remaining quantity being transferred: _____

Date of transfer: _____

Nurse/LP making transfer: _____

TRANSFER TO DIFFERENT LOCATION

New location transferred to: _____

New page number transferred to: _____

Remaining quantity being transferred: _____

Date of transfer: _____

Nurse/LP making transfer: _____

Nurse/LP receiving transfer: _____

SURRENDER TO PERSON

Remaining quantity being surrendered: _____

Nurse/LP making surrender: _____

Person Surrendered To
Printed Name: _____
Signature: _____
- Patient - Responsible Party - Nurse/LP - Administrator - (circle one)

DEPLETION OF DRUG / MED
NONE REMAINING – PAGE FINISHED

Date completed: _____

Nurse/LP completing: _____

CONTROLLED DRUG / MED SUPPLY

Drug / Med Name:

Drug / Med Given			Present Balance	In From Pharmacy	Patient's Name	Prescriber's Name	Nurse/LP's Signature
Date	Time	Dose					

Two Nurse/LPs must witness and sign the destruction / waste of any controlled drugs / meds.
When folding pages over, the disposition of drugs / meds must be documented appropriately.

CONTROLLED DRUG / MED DISPOSITION

The applicable box below must be completed
when this page is folded over.

TRANSFER TO NEW PAGE

New page number transferred to: _____

Remaining quantity being transferred: _____

Date of transfer: _____

Nurse/LP making transfer: _____

TRANSFER TO DIFFERENT LOCATION

New location transferred to: _____

New page number transferred to: _____

Remaining quantity being transferred: _____

Date of transfer: _____

Nurse/LP making transfer: _____

Nurse/LP receiving transfer: _____

SURRENDER TO PERSON

Remaining quantity being surrendered: _____

Nurse/LP making surrender: _____

Person Surrendered To
Printed Name: _____
Signature: _____
- Patient - Responsible Party - Nurse/LP - Administrator - (circle one)

DEPLETION OF DRUG / MED
NONE REMAINING – PAGE FINISHED

Date completed: _____

Nurse/LP completing: _____

CONTROLLED DRUG / MED SUPPLY

Drug / Med Name: Page No: **137**

Drug / Med Given			Present Balance	In From Pharmacy	Patient's Name	Prescriber's Name	Nurse/LP's Signature
Date	Time	Dose					

Two Nurse/LPs must witness and sign the destruction / waste of any controlled drugs / meds.
When folding pages over, the disposition of drugs / meds must be documented appropriately.

CONTROLLED DRUG / MED DISPOSITION

The applicable box below must be completed when this page is folded over.

TRANSFER TO NEW PAGE

New page number transferred to: _____

Remaining quantity being transferred: _____

Date of transfer: _____

Nurse/LP making transfer: _____

TRANSFER TO DIFFERENT LOCATION

New location transferred to: _____

New page number transferred to: _____

Remaining quantity being transferred: _____

Date of transfer: _____

Nurse/LP making transfer: _____

Nurse/LP receiving transfer: _____

SURRENDER TO PERSON

Remaining quantity being surrendered: _____

Nurse/LP making surrender: _____

Person Surrendered To
Printed Name: _____
Signature: _____
- Patient - Responsible Party - Nurse/LP - Administrator -   (circle one)

DEPLETION OF DRUG / MED
NONE REMAINING – PAGE FINISHED

Date completed: _____

Nurse/LP completing: _____

CONTROLLED DRUG / MED SUPPLY

Drug / Med Name:

Drug / Med Given			Present Balance	In From Pharmacy	Patient's Name	Prescriber's Name	Nurse/LP's Signature
Date	Time	Dose					

Two Nurse/LPs must witness and sign the destruction / waste of any controlled drugs / meds.
When folding pages over, the disposition of drugs / meds must be documented appropriately.

CONTROLLED DRUG / MED DISPOSITION

*The applicable box below must be completed
when this page is folded over.*

TRANSFER TO NEW PAGE

New page number transferred to: _____

Remaining quantity being transferred: _____

Date of transfer: _____

Nurse/LP making transfer: _____

TRANSFER TO DIFFERENT LOCATION

New location transferred to: _____

New page number transferred to: _____

Remaining quantity being transferred: _____

Date of transfer: _____

Nurse/LP making transfer: _____

Nurse/LP receiving transfer: _____

SURRENDER TO PERSON

Remaining quantity being surrendered: _____

Nurse/LP making surrender: _____

Person Surrendered To
Printed Name: _____
Signature: _____
- Patient - Responsible Party - Nurse/LP - Administrator - (circle one)

DEPLETION OF DRUG / MED
NONE REMAINING – PAGE FINISHED

Date completed: _____

Nurse/LP completing: _____

CONTROLLED DRUG / MED SUPPLY

Drug / Med Name: ⠀⠀⠀⠀⠀⠀⠀⠀⠀⠀⠀⠀⠀⠀⠀⠀Page No: **139**

Drug / Med Given			Present Balance	In From Pharmacy	Patient's Name	Prescriber's Name	Nurse/LP's Signature
Date	Time	Dose					

Two Nurse/LPs must witness and sign the destruction / waste of any controlled drugs / meds.
When folding pages over, the disposition of drugs / meds must be documented appropriately.

CONTROLLED DRUG / MED DISPOSITION

The applicable box below must be completed
when this page is folded over.

TRANSFER TO NEW PAGE

New page number transferred to: _____

Remaining quantity being transferred: _____

Date of transfer: _____

Nurse/LP making transfer: _____

TRANSFER TO DIFFERENT LOCATION

New location transferred to: _____

New page number transferred to: _____

Remaining quantity being transferred: _____

Date of transfer: _____

Nurse/LP making transfer: _____

Nurse/LP receiving transfer: _____

SURRENDER TO PERSON

Remaining quantity being surrendered: _____

Nurse/LP making surrender: _____

Person Surrendered To
Printed Name: _____
Signature: _____
- Patient - Responsible Party - Nurse/LP - Administrator - (circle one)

DEPLETION OF DRUG / MED
NONE REMAINING – PAGE FINISHED

Date completed: _____

Nurse/LP completing: _____

CONTROLLED DRUG / MED SUPPLY

Drug / Med Name:

Drug / Med Given			Present Balance	In From Pharmacy	Patient's Name	Prescriber's Name	Nurse/LP's Signature
Date	Time	Dose					

Two Nurse/LPs must witness and sign the destruction / waste of any controlled drugs / meds.
When folding pages over, the disposition of drugs / meds must be documented appropriately.

CONTROLLED DRUG / MED DISPOSITION

*The applicable box below must be completed
when this page is folded over.*

TRANSFER TO NEW PAGE

New page number transferred to: _____

Remaining quantity being transferred: _____

Date of transfer: _____

Nurse/LP making transfer: _____

TRANSFER TO DIFFERENT LOCATION

New location transferred to: _____

New page number transferred to: _____

Remaining quantity being transferred: _____

Date of transfer: _____

Nurse/LP making transfer: _____

Nurse/LP receiving transfer: _____

SURRENDER TO PERSON

Remaining quantity being surrendered: _____

Nurse/LP making surrender: _____

Person Surrendered To
Printed Name: _____
Signature: _____
- Patient - Responsible Party - Nurse/LP - Administrator - (circle one)

DEPLETION OF DRUG / MED
NONE REMAINING – PAGE FINISHED

Date completed: _____

Nurse/LP completing: _____

CONTROLLED DRUG / MED SUPPLY

Drug / Med Name: Page No: **141**

Drug / Med Given			Present Balance	In From Pharmacy	Patient's Name	Prescriber's Name	Nurse/LP's Signature
Date	Time	Dose					

Two Nurse/LPs must witness and sign the destruction / waste of any controlled drugs / meds.
When folding pages over, the disposition of drugs / meds must be documented appropriately.

CONTROLLED DRUG / MED DISPOSITION

*The applicable box below must be completed
when this page is folded over.*

TRANSFER TO NEW PAGE

New page number transferred to: _____

Remaining quantity being transferred: _____

Date of transfer: _____

Nurse/LP making transfer: _____

TRANSFER TO DIFFERENT LOCATION

New location transferred to: _____

New page number transferred to: _____

Remaining quantity being transferred: _____

Date of transfer: _____

Nurse/LP making transfer: _____

Nurse/LP receiving transfer: _____

SURRENDER TO PERSON

Remaining quantity being surrendered: _____

Nurse/LP making surrender: _____

Person Surrendered To
Printed Name: _____
Signature: _____
- Patient - Responsible Party - Nurse/LP - Administrator - (circle one)

DEPLETION OF DRUG / MED
NONE REMAINING – PAGE FINISHED

Date completed: _____

Nurse/LP completing: _____

CONTROLLED DRUG / MED SUPPLY

Drug / Med Name: Page No: **142**

Drug / Med Given			Present Balance	In From Pharmacy	Patient's Name	Prescriber's Name	Nurse/LP's Signature
Date	Time	Dose					

Two Nurse/LPs must witness and sign the destruction / waste of any controlled drugs / meds.
When folding pages over, the disposition of drugs / meds must be documented appropriately.

CONTROLLED DRUG / MED DISPOSITION

The applicable box below must be completed
when this page is folded over.

TRANSFER TO NEW PAGE

New page number transferred to: _____

Remaining quantity being transferred: _____

Date of transfer: _____

Nurse/LP making transfer: _____

TRANSFER TO DIFFERENT LOCATION

New location transferred to: _____

New page number transferred to: _____

Remaining quantity being transferred: _____

Date of transfer: _____

Nurse/LP making transfer: _____

Nurse/LP receiving transfer: _____

SURRENDER TO PERSON

Remaining quantity being surrendered: _____

Nurse/LP making surrender: _____

Person Surrendered To
Printed Name: _____
Signature: _____
- Patient - Responsible Party - Nurse/LP - Administrator - (circle one)

DEPLETION OF DRUG / MED
NONE REMAINING – PAGE FINISHED

Date completed: _____

Nurse/LP completing: _____

CONTROLLED DRUG / MED SUPPLY

Drug / Med Name: Page No: **143**

Drug / Med Given			Present Balance	In From Pharmacy	Patient's Name	Prescriber's Name	Nurse/LP's Signature
Date	Time	Dose					

Two Nurse/LPs must witness and sign the destruction / waste of any controlled drugs / meds.
When folding pages over, the disposition of drugs / meds must be documented appropriately.

CONTROLLED DRUG / MED DISPOSITION

The applicable box below must be completed
when this page is folded over.

TRANSFER TO NEW PAGE

New page number transferred to: _____

Remaining quantity being transferred: _____

Date of transfer: _____

Nurse/LP making transfer: _____

TRANSFER TO DIFFERENT LOCATION

New location transferred to: _____

New page number transferred to: _____

Remaining quantity being transferred: _____

Date of transfer: _____

Nurse/LP making transfer: _____

Nurse/LP receiving transfer: _____

SURRENDER TO PERSON

Remaining quantity being surrendered: _____

Nurse/LP making surrender: _____

Person Surrendered To
Printed Name: _____
Signature: _____
- Patient - Responsible Party - Nurse/LP - Administrator - (circle one)

DEPLETION OF DRUG / MED
NONE REMAINING – PAGE FINISHED

Date completed: _____

Nurse/LP completing: _____

CONTROLLED DRUG / MED SUPPLY

Drug / Med Name: Page No: **144**

Drug / Med Given			Present Balance	In From Pharmacy	Patient's Name	Prescriber's Name	Nurse/LP's Signature
Date	Time	Dose					

Two Nurse/LPs must witness and sign the destruction / waste of any controlled drugs / meds.
When folding pages over, the disposition of drugs / meds must be documented appropriately.

CONTROLLED DRUG / MED DISPOSITION

*The applicable box below must be completed
when this page is folded over.*

TRANSFER TO NEW PAGE

New page number transferred to: _____

Remaining quantity being transferred: _____

Date of transfer: _____

Nurse/LP making transfer: _____

TRANSFER TO DIFFERENT LOCATION

New location transferred to: _____

New page number transferred to: _____

Remaining quantity being transferred: _____

Date of transfer: _____

Nurse/LP making transfer: _____

Nurse/LP receiving transfer: _____

SURRENDER TO PERSON

Remaining quantity being surrendered: _____

Nurse/LP making surrender: _____

Person Surrendered To
Printed Name: _____
Signature: _____
- Patient - Responsible Party - Nurse/LP - Administrator - (circle one)

DEPLETION OF DRUG / MED
NONE REMAINING – PAGE FINISHED

Date completed: _____

Nurse/LP completing: _____

CONTROLLED DRUG / MED SUPPLY

Drug / Med Name: Page No: **145**

Drug / Med Given			Present Balance	In From Pharmacy	Patient's Name	Prescriber's Name	Nurse/LP's Signature
Date	Time	Dose					

Two Nurse/LPs must witness and sign the destruction / waste of any controlled drugs / meds.
When folding pages over, the disposition of drugs / meds must be documented appropriately.

CONTROLLED DRUG / MED DISPOSITION

The applicable box below must be completed
when this page is folded over.

TRANSFER TO NEW PAGE

New page number transferred to: _____

Remaining quantity being transferred: _____

Date of transfer: _____

Nurse/LP making transfer: _____

TRANSFER TO DIFFERENT LOCATION

New location transferred to: _____

New page number transferred to: _____

Remaining quantity being transferred: _____

Date of transfer: _____

Nurse/LP making transfer: _____

Nurse/LP receiving transfer: _____

SURRENDER TO PERSON

Remaining quantity being surrendered: _____

Nurse/LP making surrender: _____

Person Surrendered To
Printed Name: _____
Signature: _____
- Patient - Responsible Party - Nurse/LP - Administrator - (circle one)

DEPLETION OF DRUG / MED
NONE REMAINING – PAGE FINISHED

Date completed: _____

Nurse/LP completing: _____

CONTROLLED DRUG / MED SUPPLY

Drug / Med Name: _____   Page No: **146**

Drug / Med Given			Present Balance	In From Pharmacy	Patient's Name	Prescriber's Name	Nurse/LP's Signature
Date	Time	Dose					

Two Nurse/LPs must witness and sign the destruction / waste of any controlled drugs / meds.
When folding pages over, the disposition of drugs / meds must be documented appropriately.

CONTROLLED DRUG / MED DISPOSITION

The applicable box below must be completed
when this page is folded over.

TRANSFER TO NEW PAGE

New page number transferred to: _____

Remaining quantity being transferred: _____

Date of transfer: _____

Nurse/LP making transfer: _____

TRANSFER TO DIFFERENT LOCATION

New location transferred to: _____

New page number transferred to: _____

Remaining quantity being transferred: _____

Date of transfer: _____

Nurse/LP making transfer: _____

Nurse/LP receiving transfer: _____

SURRENDER TO PERSON

Remaining quantity being surrendered: _____

Nurse/LP making surrender: _____

Person Surrendered To
Printed Name: _____
Signature: _____
- Patient - Responsible Party - Nurse/LP - Administrator - (circle one)

DEPLETION OF DRUG / MED
NONE REMAINING – PAGE FINISHED

Date completed: _____

Nurse/LP completing: _____

CONTROLLED DRUG / MED SUPPLY

Drug / Med Name: Page No: **147**

Drug / Med Given			Present Balance	In From Pharmacy	Patient's Name	Prescriber's Name	Nurse/LP's Signature
Date	Time	Dose					

Two Nurse/LPs must witness and sign the destruction / waste of any controlled drugs / meds.
When folding pages over, the disposition of drugs / meds must be documented appropriately.

CONTROLLED DRUG / MED DISPOSITION

The applicable box below must be completed
when this page is folded over.

TRANSFER TO NEW PAGE

New page number transferred to: _____

Remaining quantity being transferred: _____

Date of transfer: _____

Nurse/LP making transfer: _____

TRANSFER TO DIFFERENT LOCATION

New location transferred to: _____

New page number transferred to: _____

Remaining quantity being transferred: _____

Date of transfer: _____

Nurse/LP making transfer: _____

Nurse/LP receiving transfer: _____

SURRENDER TO PERSON

Remaining quantity being surrendered: _____

Nurse/LP making surrender: _____

Person Surrendered To
Printed Name: _____
Signature: _____
- Patient - Responsible Party - Nurse/LP - Administrator - (circle one)

DEPLETION OF DRUG / MED
NONE REMAINING – PAGE FINISHED

Date completed: _____

Nurse/LP completing: _____

CONTROLLED DRUG / MED SUPPLY

Drug / Med Name: Page No: **148**

Drug / Med Given			Present Balance	In From Pharmacy	Patient's Name	Prescriber's Name	Nurse/LP's Signature
Date	Time	Dose					

Two Nurse/LPs must witness and sign the destruction / waste of any controlled drugs / meds.
When folding pages over, the disposition of drugs / meds must be documented appropriately.

CONTROLLED DRUG / MED DISPOSITION

The applicable box below must be completed
when this page is folded over.

TRANSFER TO NEW PAGE

New page number transferred to: _____

Remaining quantity being transferred: _____

Date of transfer: _____

Nurse/LP making transfer: _____

TRANSFER TO DIFFERENT LOCATION

New location transferred to: _____

New page number transferred to: _____

Remaining quantity being transferred: _____

Date of transfer: _____

Nurse/LP making transfer: _____

Nurse/LP receiving transfer: _____

SURRENDER TO PERSON

Remaining quantity being surrendered: _____

Nurse/LP making surrender: _____

Person Surrendered To
Printed Name: _____
Signature: _____
- Patient - Responsible Party - Nurse/LP - Administrator - (circle one)

DEPLETION OF DRUG / MED
NONE REMAINING – PAGE FINISHED

Date completed: _____

Nurse/LP completing: _____

CONTROLLED DRUG / MED SUPPLY

Drug / Med Name: Page No: **149**

Drug / Med Given			Present Balance	In From Pharmacy	Patient's Name	Prescriber's Name	Nurse/LP's Signature
Date	Time	Dose					

Two Nurse/LPs must witness and sign the destruction / waste of any controlled drugs / meds.
When folding pages over, the disposition of drugs / meds must be documented appropriately.

CONTROLLED DRUG / MED DISPOSITION

*The applicable box below must be completed
when this page is folded over.*

TRANSFER TO NEW PAGE

New page number transferred to: _____

Remaining quantity being transferred: _____

Date of transfer: _____

Nurse/LP making transfer: _____

TRANSFER TO DIFFERENT LOCATION

New location transferred to: _____

New page number transferred to: _____

Remaining quantity being transferred: _____

Date of transfer: _____

Nurse/LP making transfer: _____

Nurse/LP receiving transfer: _____

SURRENDER TO PERSON

Remaining quantity being surrendered: _____

Nurse/LP making surrender: _____

Person Surrendered To
Printed Name: _____
Signature: _____
- Patient - Responsible Party - Nurse/LP - Administrator - (circle one)

DEPLETION OF DRUG / MED
NONE REMAINING – PAGE FINISHED

Date completed: _____

Nurse/LP completing: _____

CONTROLLED DRUG / MED SUPPLY

Drug / Med Name:

Drug / Med Given			Present Balance	In From Pharmacy	Patient's Name	Prescriber's Name	Nurse/LP's Signature
Date	Time	Dose					

Two Nurse/LPs must witness and sign the destruction / waste of any controlled drugs / meds.
When folding pages over, the disposition of drugs / meds must be documented appropriately.

CONTROLLED DRUG / MED DISPOSITION

The applicable box below must be completed
when this page is folded over.

TRANSFER TO NEW PAGE

New page number transferred to: _____

Remaining quantity being transferred: _____

Date of transfer: _____

Nurse/LP making transfer: _____

TRANSFER TO DIFFERENT LOCATION

New location transferred to: _____

New page number transferred to: _____

Remaining quantity being transferred: _____

Date of transfer: _____

Nurse/LP making transfer: _____

Nurse/LP receiving transfer: _____

SURRENDER TO PERSON

Remaining quantity being surrendered: _____

Nurse/LP making surrender: _____

Person Surrendered To
Printed Name: _____
Signature: _____
- Patient - Responsible Party - Nurse/LP - Administrator -   (circle one)

DEPLETION OF DRUG / MED
NONE REMAINING – PAGE FINISHED

Date completed: _____

Nurse/LP completing: _____

- Order Copies -

www.maxnjax.com/substancebook
email us at: info@maxnjax.com
amazon.com, using the ISBN number above
(visit our web site for special offers)

67225514R00199

Made in the USA
Middletown, DE
09 September 2019